# WANDERINGS
## A Psychiatrist Reflects on People, Places, and Health

# WANDERINGS

## A Psychiatrist Reflects on People, Places, and Health

by
**Ezra E. H. Griffith, M.D.**

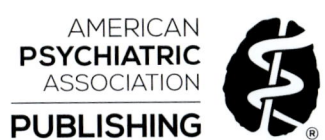

**Note:** The authors have worked to ensure that all information in this book is accurate at the time of publication and consistent with general psychiatric and medical standards, and that information concerning drug dosages, schedules, and routes of administration is accurate at the time of publication and consistent with standards set by the U.S. Food and Drug Administration and the general medical community. As medical research and practice continue to advance, however, therapeutic standards may change. Moreover, specific situations may require a specific therapeutic response not included in this book. For these reasons and because human and mechanical errors sometimes occur, we recommend that readers follow the advice of physicians directly involved in their care or the care of a member of their family.

Books published by American Psychiatric Association Publishing represent the findings, conclusions, and views of the individual authors and do not necessarily represent the policies and opinions of American Psychiatric Association Publishing or the American Psychiatric Association.

Copyright © 2025 American Psychiatric Association.
ALL RIGHTS RESERVED.

Unless authorized in writing by the APA, no part of this book may be reproduced or used in a manner inconsistent with APA's copyright. This prohibition applies to unauthorized uses or reproductions in any form, including electronic applications. For inquiries about permissions or licensing, please contact the Permissions and Licensing department at the address below or submit inquiries online at www.appi.org/Support/Customer-Information/Permissions.

If you wish to buy 50 or more copies of the same title, please visit www.appi.org/specialdiscounts for more information.

First Edition
Manufactured in the United States of America on acid-free paper
29  28  27  26  25    5  4  3  2  1

American Psychiatric Association Publishing
800 Maine Avenue SW, Suite 900
Washington, DC 20024-2812
www.appi.org

**Library of Congress Cataloging-in-Publication Data**
Names: Griffith, Ezra E. H., 1942- author.
Title: Wanderings : a psychiatrist reflects on people, places, and health / Ezra E.H. Griffith, M.D.
Other titles: Psychiatric news.
Description: Third edition. | Washington, DC : American Psychiatric Association Publishing, [2025] | Previously published columns from Psychiatric News. | Includes bibliographical references and index.
Identifiers: LCCN 2025027828 (print) | LCCN 2025027829 (ebook) | ISBN 9798894551401 (paperback) | ISBN 9798894551418 (ebook)
Subjects: LCSH: Social psychiatry. | Interpersonal relations.
Classification: LCC RC455 .G75 2025 (print) | LCC RC455 (ebook)
LC record available at https://lccn.loc.gov/2025027828
LC ebook record available at https://lccn.loc.gov/2025027829

**British Library Cataloguing in Publication Data**
A CIP record is available from the British Library.

**EU GPSR Authorized Representative: LOGOS EUROPE**, 9 rue Nicolas Poussin, 17000, LA ROCHELLE, France; email: Contact@logoseurope.eu

# Contents

About the Author . . . . . . . . . . . . . . . . . . . . . . . . xi

Acknowledgments . . . . . . . . . . . . . . . . . . . . . . . xiii

Foreword: Building Theory and Practice
From Our Backgrounds . . . . . . . . . . . . . . . . xv

    Portraiture as a Method . . . . . . . . . . . . . . . . . . . xviii

    Interrogating the Relationship Between
        Place and Culture . . . . . . . . . . . . . . . . . . . . . . . xix

    Immigration's Effects on Developmental
        Psychology . . . . . . . . . . . . . . . . . . . . . . . . . . . . xxi

    Culture and Meaning-Making
        Across Identities . . . . . . . . . . . . . . . . . . . . . . . . xxii

Introduction: On the Making of This Text . . xxvii

    Background . . . . . . . . . . . . . . . . . . . . . . . . . . . . . xxvii

    Change in the Air . . . . . . . . . . . . . . . . . . . . . . . . xxviii

    Envisioning the Book . . . . . . . . . . . . . . . . . . . . . . xxix

    Race Matters . . . . . . . . . . . . . . . . . . . . . . . . . . . . . xxxi

    Centrality of Place . . . . . . . . . . . . . . . . . . . . . . . . xxxii

    Biography and Narrative . . . . . . . . . . . . . . . . . . xxxiii

    Audience and Structure . . . . . . . . . . . . . . . . . . . xxxiv

# 1 Considering Race Matters . . . . . . . . . . . . . . . 1

## Columns From *Psychiatric News* . . . . . . . . . . . . . . . . 2
### When Diversity Is Not Enough... . . . . . . . . . . . . . . . . . . . . 2
### Black Identity Politics and Psychiatry . . . . . . . . . . . . . . . . . 4
### Hate in the Context of Oppression . . . . . . . . . . . . . . . . . . . 6
### On Caste and Suffering... . . . . . . . . . . . . . . . . . . . . . . . . . . 8
### The Knee on the Other's Neck... . . . . . . . . . . . . . . . . . . . 10
### Diversity and Curiosity About the Other... . . . . . . . . . . . 16
### Talking About Freedom With Louis Menand . . . . . . . . . . . 17

## Comments and Clinical Observations . . . . . . . . . . 21

## Questions to Ponder . . . . . . . . . . . . . . . . . . . . . . . 28

# 2 Pursuing Dignity . . . . . . . . . . . . . . . . . . . . . 31

## Columns From *Psychiatric News* . . . . . . . . . . . . . . . . 32
### Empathy, Compassion, and Dignity in
### Forensic Psychiatry . . . . . . . . . . . . . . . . . . . . . . . . . . . 32
### Memorializing Dignity and Identity in
### Public Monuments... . . . . . . . . . . . . . . . . . . . . . . . . 34
### Identity and Political Independence . . . . . . . . . . . . . . . . . 37
### The Justice and Affirmative Action... . . . . . . . . . . . . . . . 39
### Expanding the Limits of Empathy... . . . . . . . . . . . . . . . . 40
### Making Choices on a Journey . . . . . . . . . . . . . . . . . . . . . 42
### The Long Journey From Arigbawonwo... . . . . . . . . . . . . . 45
### When Outsiders Come In . . . . . . . . . . . . . . . . . . . . . . . . 48
### That Music From Overseas... . . . . . . . . . . . . . . . . . . . . . 51

## Comments and Clinical Observations . . . . . . . . . . 53

## Questions to Ponder . . . . . . . . . . . . . . . . . . . . . . . 61

# 3 Facing Disability . . . . . . . . . . . . . . . . . . . . . . 63

## Columns From *Psychiatric News* . . . . . . . . . . . . . . 64
*The Silence of the Deaf . . . . . . . . . . . . . . . . . . . . . . . . . . . . . 64*
*Reply to Larry Davidson on Recovery . . . . . . . . . . . . . . . 65*
*Creative Writing and Psychiatric Rehabilitation . . . . . . . . . 67*
*'Homes' at the Sainte-Anne Hospital Museum . . . . . . . . . 69*
*Memories of a Community Hospital . . . . . . . . . . . . . . . . . 72*
*Seeing the World Through Writers' Eyes . . . . . . . . . . . . . . 76*
*End-of-Year Rituals and New Year Promises . . . . . . . . . . . 78*
*Reflecting on Forgiveness . . . . . . . . . . . . . . . . . . . . . . . . . 80*
*Francesc Tosquelles and the Art of*
  *Institutional Psychotherapy . . . . . . . . . . . . . . . . . . . . . 83*

## Comments and Clinical Observations . . . . . . . . . 87

## Questions to Ponder . . . . . . . . . . . . . . . . . . . . . . 94

# 4 Confronting the COVID-19 Pandemic . . . . 97

## Columns From *Psychiatric News* . . . . . . . . . . . . . . 98
*Building Community: We Gatherin' Barbados . . . . . . . . . . 98*
*My Fable of Contagion . . . . . . . . . . . . . . . . . . . . . . . . . . 100*
*Expressions of Loss and Hope . . . . . . . . . . . . . . . . . . . . . 103*
*Contemplating Changes From a Transformative Year . . . . 105*
*Angels and the Pandemic . . . . . . . . . . . . . . . . . . . . . . . . 107*
*Welcome Happy Morning . . . . . . . . . . . . . . . . . . . . . . . . 108*
*Disguising War's Misery . . . . . . . . . . . . . . . . . . . . . . . . . 111*

## Comments and Clinical Observations . . . . . . . . . 114

## Questions to Ponder . . . . . . . . . . . . . . . . . . . . . . 120

# 5 Talking About Sacred Spaces . . . . . . . . . 121

## Columns From *Psychiatric News* . . . . . . . . . . . . . 122
*Healing at the Isenheim Altarpiece . . . . . . . . . . . . . . . . . . . . 122*
*The Steel Pan and Decolonizing Mental Health . . . . . . . . 124*
*Peace Cranes in a Sanctuary . . . . . . . . . . . . . . . . . . . . . . . . 126*
*On Difference and Othering . . . . . . . . . . . . . . . . . . . . . . . . 129*
*The Pleasure of Chance Encounters . . . . . . . . . . . . . . . . . . 131*
*Exploring My Connections to Prague . . . . . . . . . . . . . . . . 134*
*A Migrant Amidst Mantuan Opulence . . . . . . . . . . . . . . . 138*
*When Africa and Europe Meet in Church . . . . . . . . . . . . 142*

## Comments and Clinical Observations . . . . . . . . . 145

## Questions to Ponder . . . . . . . . . . . . . . . . . . . . . . 151

# 6 Focusing on Place . . . . . . . . . . . . . . . . . . 153

## Columns From *Psychiatric News* . . . . . . . . . . . . . 154
*Celebrating Psychiatric Health and Place . . . . . . . . . . . . . 154*
*Lingering in a Garden . . . . . . . . . . . . . . . . . . . . . . . . . . . . 156*
*The House by the Sea . . . . . . . . . . . . . . . . . . . . . . . . . . . . 158*
*C.L.R. James' Beyond a Boundary . . . . . . . . . . . . . . . . . . 160*
*An Afternoon Constitutional . . . . . . . . . . . . . . . . . . . . . . 162*
*Archiving Our Pasts . . . . . . . . . . . . . . . . . . . . . . . . . . . . . 165*
*On Radishes and Other Culinary Memories . . . . . . . . . . 170*
*Photography as a Mirror With Memory . . . . . . . . . . . . . . 172*
*Dreaming With Freud . . . . . . . . . . . . . . . . . . . . . . . . . . . 175*
*Aging and Political Theater . . . . . . . . . . . . . . . . . . . . . . . 177*

## Comments and Clinical Observations . . . . . . . . . 180

## Questions to Ponder . . . . . . . . . . . . . . . . . . . . . . 184

# 7 Seeking Freedom Through the Arts . . . . . 185

## Columns From *Psychiatric News* . . . . . . . . . . . . . 186
Visibility in a Psychiatric Hospital's Museum. . . . . . . . . . 186
Stress in Athletes' Lives . . . . . . . . . . . . . . . . . . . . . . . . . 189
A Flamenco Tale in Edinburgh:
   Recreating Home . . . . . . . . . . . . . . . . . . . . . . . . . . . 190
Yonder on the Other Side . . . . . . . . . . . . . . . . . . . . . . . 193
The Solitude of an Artist . . . . . . . . . . . . . . . . . . . . . . . . 196
Seeking Nirvana at the Potter's Wheel . . . . . . . . . . . . . . 198
Ancestral Dignity in Public Monuments . . . . . . . . . . . . . 201
Talkin' 'Bout Harlem . . . . . . . . . . . . . . . . . . . . . . . . . . . 204
Suzanne Césaire and Caribbean Identity . . . . . . . . . . . . 207

## Comments and Clinical Observations . . . . . . . . 210

## Questions to Ponder . . . . . . . . . . . . . . . . . . . . . 216

# Epilogue . . . . . . . . . . . . . . . . . . . . . . . . . . . 217

# Index . . . . . . . . . . . . . . . . . . . . . . . . . . . . . 219

# About the Author

Ezra E. H. Griffith, M.D., is Professor Emeritus of Psychiatry and African American Studies at Yale University in New Haven, Connecticut. He earned his Bachelor of Arts degree from Harvard University and his medical degree from the University of Strasbourg Faculty of Medicine in France. In 2001, the Morehouse School of Medicine conferred on him the honorary degree Doctor of Science. Dr. Griffith has published widely in the subdisciplines of forensic psychiatry and cultural psychiatry, including approximately 200 academic articles, chapters, and commentaries and 13 books. He has written most recently on ethics and performative narrative. He has proposed human dignity as a significant factor in rendering social spaces more therapeutic. He is the editor of *Ethics Challenges in Forensic Psychiatry and Psychology Practice* (Columbia University Press, 2018) and author of *Belonging, Therapeutic Landscapes, and Networks* (Routledge, 2018) and *Race and Excellence: My Dialogue With Chester Pierce* (American Psychiatric Association Publishing, 2023). He is a coeditor of *Black Mental Health* (American Psychiatric Association Publishing, 2019).

Dr. Griffith has no affiliations or interests that may present competing interests to declare.

# Acknowledgments

Writing a book is a major task, full of problems and pitfalls. Doing it alone, truly alone, is unnecessarily burdensome. It is always a bit easier, and much more pleasant, to benefit from support, help, and encouragement. I mention several individuals who stood by me and facilitated the completion of the work. They are Brigitte Pierrette Griffith, a first-class adviser on many levels who understands photography and aesthetics; Ronald C. Grantham, AIA, who designed the beautiful cover of this book and provided several photographs; Cathy Brown, an American Psychiatric Association (APA) colleague who regularly discussed my ideas and prose; Erika Parker, acquisitions editor at APA Publishing, whose guidance was always thoughtful and constructive; and Neil K. Aggarwal, M.D., M.A., who debated my ideas and authored an insightful foreword for all to read. These individuals deserve my earnest thanks.

# Foreword: Building Theory and Practice From Our Backgrounds

I first met Ezra Griffith in 2006 while interviewing for psychiatric residency training positions. He was the deputy chair for diversity and organizational ethics, professor of psychiatry, and professor of African American studies at Yale University. By then, he had served as president of the American Academy of Psychiatry and the Law, the American Board of Forensic Psychiatry, the Black Psychiatrists of America, and the American Orthopsychiatric Association. His accolades were so numerous that Dr. Chester Pierce, an African American tenured professor of education and psychiatry at Harvard Medical School who helped to pioneer the critical study of race and racism within psychiatry, wrote the following in 1997 about Ezra:

> From all over the world, he is called on as a lecturer and consultant. The list of private and public universities, agencies, foundations, and professional and learned societies that have made this call is too long to recite in detail. Among the calls Ezra has answered have been summons to give distinguished lectures (e.g., to the American Psychiatric Association); to serve as an external examiner (e.g., at the University of the West Indies); to advise on world health issues (e.g., for the Pan American Health Organization); to be a visiting professor, particularly at law schools and medical schools (e.g., the Florida State University Law School and Northwestern University Medical School); to give keynote or special lectures (e.g., to the Royal College of Psychiatrists in England); and to take part in foundation programs (e.g., as a National Fellow to the Kellogg Foundation). (Pierce 1997, p. 339)

I mention these details because Ezra is too gracious to communicate his accomplishments to you. The quote also illustrates the esteem with which towering figures in psychiatry, like Dr. Pierce, have held him. And yet, his humility is his most admirable trait. During my residency interview, he asked about my interests in psychiatry, anthropology, and South Asian studies, mentioning casually that he had combined psychiatry, anthropology, and African American studies in his career. We discovered that we read common theorists, shared outrage at the injustices that minorities face in the United States as a legacy of settler colonialism, and felt comfortable critiquing psychiatric knowledge and practices as culturally constructed compared with our biologically oriented colleagues who saw psychiatry as closer to neuroscience. At no point did he reference any of his hundreds of book chapters or articles that have appeared in the highest impact factor journals across psychiatry and psychology.

I asked Ezra what distinguished Yale from other programs. Eschewing the reservedness of other interviewers, he answered, "Someone like you is going to do social science anywhere you go. You need the biological and psychological training to be a psychiatrist. If you come here, you'll join a community of scholars." I made up my mind instantly. Program directors can infantilize residency applicants, but Ezra treated me like a younger colleague right from the start.

We met about once a quarter during my training to discuss our interests in psychiatry and anthropology over dinner. For you to understand our discussions, I'll explain some assumptions we share. Drawing on the social sciences, researchers in cultural psychiatry explore the universality versus relativity of psychopathology and healing practices, the challenges of delivering services to minoritized populations, and the analysis of psychiatric theories and practices as culturally situated (Kirmayer 2007). Social scientists within interpretive medical anthropology have provided cultural psychiatrists with theories and ethnographic methods to uncover the cultural meanings of health, illness, narratives, and patient-provider transactions (Good et al. 2010). The fourth edition of the *Diagnostic and Statistical Manual of Mental Disorders* (DSM-IV) marked the first institutional collaboration among anthropologists, psychiatrists, and psychologists, who argued that psychiatrists should complete cultural formulations with patients, reasoning that culture shapes the expression and meaning of symptoms, the diagnostic rationales for clustering symptoms together, and the interpersonal contexts for clinical work (Mezzich et al. 1999). To inquire about symptom expressions, their clinical meanings, and the validity of DSM diagnostic categories for minority patients, DSM-IV encouraged clinicians to complete an Outline for Cultural Formulation (OCF) through five domains: 1) cultural identity of the individual, 2) cultural explanations of the individual's illness, 3) cultural factors related to the psychosocial environment and levels of functioning, 4) cultural elements of the patient-clinician relationship, and 5) an overall cultural assessment for diagnosis and care (American Psychiatric Association 1994). Since 1994, however, most publications on the OCF and the subsequent DSM-5 Cultural Formulation Interview (American Psychiatric Association 2013) have focused on operationalizing "culture" rather than "formulation" because psychological schools—cognitive, behavioral, existential, psychoanalytic, and psychodynamic, just to name a few—have differed on exactly how to do a clinical formulation, which has confounded clinicians (Aggarwal 2024).

Many have viewed collaborations between anthropologists and psychiatrists with suspicion. Some anthropologists worry that medical anthropology is moving too close to medicine in incorporating, rather than critiquing, biomedical concepts. Also, practices have historically subjugated groups of people, such as women (Lock 2001). On the other side, physicians have critiqued anthropologists for too readily highlighting problems with medical systems without providing realistic solutions (Hemmings 2005). Ezra's work stands apart for taking courageous intellectual stands that demonstrate the relevance of anthropology to psychiatry. One longitudinal current throughout his work has been to examine how the forensic psychiatrist-evaluee relationship is similar to and different from the treating psychiatrist-patient relationship. He was the first in forensic psychiatry to recommend that clinicians reflect on cultural elements of the clinician-evaluee relationship, whether they belong to the same or different cultural reference groups as their evaluees (Griffith 1996), which emphasizes the importance of culture to *all* interactions, whether they are treatment-based or forensic. He introduced cultural formulations into forensic practice, showing that cultural analyses of the evaluee, their explanations of behavior, and the clinician-evaluee relationship can lead to four possible formulations of expert opinion in criminal cases: a negation of culture, a desire to advance the sociopolitical interests of White Americans, a temptation to side with minoritized populations who have been wronged in the criminal justice system, or a truthful assessment of the evaluee's experience within the psychosocial environment (Griffith 1998). Turning to the act of writing, Griffith and Madelon Baranoski (2007) have argued that forensic reports are not impersonal and objective in the experimental scientific sense because they necessarily reflect the expert's perspectives, fee arrangements, cultural identity, upbringing, and preference for working with one legal side over another. And in probing why courtroom testimony is "informative and performative," Griffith and Baranoski (2011) have drawn on ritual theory in anthropology to delineate stages in the expert witness's performance: making a grand entrance into court, initiating the performance through the establishment of credentials, using storytelling to narrate the expert opinion, withstanding cross-examination, and the finale.

Ezra envisions culture as essential to the clinician's core tasks of interviewing, writing, and testifying. Mixing rigorous analyses of scholarship across several disciplines with critical reflections on his identity, Ezra reminds us repeatedly that we all need to accept the uncomfortable truth that our positions in the social world influence our authoritative interpretations of others' behaviors. This social fact helps to explain his preoccupation with elaborating a professional ethics that honors, rather than ignores, our real-world commitments. I interpret Ezra's body of work as pushing cultural psychiatrists to think practically about the implications that demographic differences—based on ethnicity, gender identity, race, and sexual orientation, just to name a few—have in society, with specific applications to the law. In retirement, Ezra continues to write, mentor, and present at scientific conferences. Now that I have caught you up on our dialogue over the past 17 years and why I hold him in such esteem, I use my space to highlight academic themes in this book. My intent is not to serve as his interpreter—his work speaks resolutely for itself—but to expand our colloquy to include readers.

## Portraiture as a Method

Ezra Griffith and Madelon Baranoski (2007) have used the work of Sara Lawrence-Lightfoot and Jessica Davis (1997) to ponder how forensic psychiatrists could portray evaluees in their reports. Lawrence-Lightfoot and Davis (1997, p. xv) have written:

> Portraiture is a method of qualitative research that blurs the boundaries of aesthetics and empiricism in an effort to capture the complexity, dynamics, and subtlety of human experience and organizational life. Portraitists seek to record and interpret the perspectives and experiences of the people they are studying, documenting their voices and their visions.

In considering the application of these ideas within a forensic context, Griffith and Baranoski (2007, p. 29) proposed:

> In using voice as a witness, the portraitist takes an outsider's stance and, like a cultural anthropologist, describes the subject of the portrait and his context from a position on the boundary of the action. However, the portraitist then goes on to use his voice in interpretation, in a search for meaning of his observations that were made as a witness from the boundary. With the voice as preoccupation, the portraitist is preoccupied with his theoretical perspectives, intellectual interests, and understanding of the relevant literature, which define the framework used by the portraitist in observations and interpretation.

I read Ezra's current book as a collection of portraits. Griffith and Baranoski have underscored that in writing (2007) and testifying (2011), psychiatrists must develop skills in observing others and themselves to develop unique, credible, convincing voices. The portraits you read continue Ezra's quest to represent others with dignity. Now, it will not surprise you when I point out that Ezra is acknowledging his intellectual debts to Lawrence-Lightfoot, a prominent African American scholar, while also drawing from anthropology in his vision for psychiatry. I would not dare attempt to psychoanalyze Ezra, but the facts suggest that Ezra, as a Black immigrant, has tried to preserve the dignity of others because he knows of the indignities that Black people face in being overrepresented in the American criminal justice system. He shows us his eagerness to traverse academic disciplines when he writes in this book that one course he taught in the Department of African American Studies "focused on studies of Black autobiographies from different social, professional, and psychological perspectives." All social scientists build theory based on lived experiences, and Ezra's goal to portray others with dignity unites his personal and professional aspirations.

## Interrogating the Relationship Between Place and Culture

Ezra's reflections on place are one of the most sustained attempts among psychiatrists to grapple with a key theoretical development in anthropology. Ezra writes in this book, "Places provide meaning for us all. For some, it includes a sense of identity, security, family life, and employment. Other times, place signifies maltreatment and indignity."

These statements recall the groundbreaking work of the anthropologists Akhil Gupta and James Ferguson (1992, pp. 6–7), who pointed out

> It is so taken for granted that each country embodies its own distinctive culture and society that the terms "society" and "culture" are routinely simply appended to the names of nation-states, as when a tourist visits India to understand "Indian culture" and "Indian society," or Thailand to experience "Thai culture," or the United States to get a whiff of "American culture."

Gupta and Ferguson (1992, p. 7) list three problems from this "isomorphism of space, place, and culture." First, it cannot account for the experience of people who inhabit borderlands, the "migrant workers, nomads, and members of the transnational business and professional elite" (p. 7), classes of people to which Ezra and I belong as third culture kids who grew up in cultural surroundings other than those of their parents (Useem and Downie 1976). Second, this isomorphism does not address intracultural variations, for Gupta and Ferguson (1992, p. 8) characterize multiculturalism as "a feeble acknowledgment of the fact that cultures have lost their moorings in definite places and an attempt to subsume this plurality of cultures within the framework of a national identity." Finally, it does not consider the realities of postcoloniality, which recur throughout Ezra's portraits. Gupta and Ferguson (1992, p. 8) pose questions that we all should contemplate: "To which places do the hybrid cultures of postcoloniality belong? Does the colonial encounter create a 'new culture' in both the colonized and colonizing countries, or does it destabilize the notion that nations and cultures are isomorphic?" Ezra's observations on the use of the Caribbean steel pan in European classical music exemplify the creation of new cultural forms born from the colonial encounter.

As a solution, Gupta and Ferguson (1992, p. 16) proposed, "A first step on this road is to move beyond naturalized conceptions of spatialized 'cultures' and to explore instead the production of difference within common, shared, and connected spaces." Ezra is the only psychiatrist I know who has publicly stepped onto this road as his portraits compel us to think about place in our production of interpersonal similarities and differences. Even if you are not an immigrant or someone at the borderlands, you probably move among homes, workplaces, and third spaces. Therefore, the idea that place influences our behaviors and the behaviors of others through forms of social conduct could complicate how we understand identity and family.

*Foreword: Building Theory and Practice From Our Backgrounds*  xxi

# Immigration's Effects on Developmental Psychology

The need to interrogate direct, simple relationships among space, place, and culture for migrants recurs in the book as Ezra excavates the cultural tributaries feeding into the stream of his identity. Born in 1942, Ezra tells us that his parents moved from Barbados to Brooklyn in 1956, that "migration was a common occurrence among West Indian families" because "employment and economic opportunities were relatively rare in the small Caribbean islands." Ezra describes the turbulence of migration: "Movement north to New York rendered everything precarious, and it transformed identity into a tool that was frail and always dependent on the support of others. That external aid was mercifully there, from friends, church, relatives, and other unlikely sources." Ezra also names the anchors that oriented him in the United States: "My buddies and I also flocked after school to the homeroom of a biology teacher who had Caribbean parents. The school ambience felt good, comfortable. The daily rhythms were predictable and enjoyable."

These experiences provide a first-person account of the immigrant adolescent's journey into adulthood. As the psychologist Anne K. Reitz writes with colleagues:

> Adolescence is a particularly taxing transitional phase, because individuals are expected to prepare for adult roles in society and to function in their social environments, including managing enlarged peer networks and academic demands.… Because immigrant adolescents grow up in at least two cultures, they face another core task, namely acculturation. Acculturation is the process of cultural and psychological change that takes place following continuous cultural contact and involves behaviors, attitudes, and values. (Reitz et al. 2014, p. 755)

The detail of flocking to the homeroom of a teacher with Caribbean origins with friends shows us how the adolescent Ezra met these developmental tasks of consolidating peer networks, meeting academic tasks, and acculturating into the United States while finding role models who shared elements of his heritage. Ezra's life mirrors demographic changes in the psychiatric workforce. International medical graduates constitute 29% of active psychiatrists and 21% of psychiatry residents in the United States (Duvivier et al. 2022). Ezra also shares portraits of immigrant physicians in the book. I wonder how we could collectively reimagine a science of developmental psychology that takes seriously the reality that in a globalized world, many of us accomplish developmental and acculturative tasks simultaneously.

# Culture and Meaning-Making Across Identities

Ezra and I see issues of culture, diversity, equity, and representation similarly. I provide my view here, which is relevant to academic medicine as a whole and psychiatry in particular.

Let's start with the idea of culture as an intersubjective process. After surveying the history of psychiatry's research on colonized populations, the psychiatrist-anthropologist Roland Littlewood (1996, p. 245) has written, "In its attempt to become recognised as a purely naturalistic science, independent of the particular moral values in which it has developed, Western medicine has played down the social relationship between patient and doctor." Indeed, the history of cultural competence movements demonstrates that from the 1970s through the 2000s, clinicians conceptualized culture as a phenomenon belonging to minority patients, typically manifested in explanations of illness or treatment preferences that inconveniently did not correspond with medical science (Aggarwal 2023). But psychoanalytic theories challenge the premise of patients and clinicians as separate entities. Instead, many of us view cross-cultural interactions through intersubjectivity—that is, patients and clinicians have distinct identities, but we all find ways to relate to one another's age, race, ethnicity, gender, sexual orientation, geographic origin, and other characteristics (Aggarwal 2011). I do not want to get lost in the details of defining culture here because my more fundamental point is that culture is not a possession to be had but a process through which all of us make meanings with one another.

As clinicians and social scientists, Ezra and I know that the doctor-patient relationship is not among equals but among people with different statuses in power. I want to connect Gupta and Ferguson's (1992) encouragement to explore the production of difference within shared spaces to the trailblazing work of Kimberlé Crenshaw and other legal scholars who have advanced our understanding of identities as being "intersectional" across demographic categories. They wrote:

> What makes an analysis intersectional—whatever terms it deploys, whatever its iteration, whatever its field or discipline—is its adoption of an intersectional way of thinking about the problem of sameness

and difference and its relation to power. This framing—conceiving of categories not as distinct but as always permeated by other categories, fluid and changing, always in the process of creating and being created by dynamics of power—emphasizes what intersectionality does rather than what intersectionality is. Thus, as conversations about intersectionality traverse the disciplines of women's/gender/feminist studies, critical race studies, and women-of-color feminism in a centripetal fashion, we would hope that bridges will continue to be built into the centrifugal forces of intersectionality. (Cho et al. 2013, p. 795)

From this perspective, Ezra and I both believe that diversity and representation are not sufficient goals for professional medical organizations and universities. In fact, we share the view that respectful dialogues alone will not get us to equality without pinpointing the reasons for power imbalances and proposing solutions that redistribute power to historically disadvantaged groups. As a professor at Columbia University who is affiliated with the New York State Center of Excellence for Cultural Competence, I hear administrators readily and trendily virtue signal about diversity and inclusion. But they are unprepared to commit salaries, benefits, and leadership positions to people of color. Like female psychiatrists from racial and ethnic minority backgrounds (Jordan et al. 2021), I have expended labor by teaching, supervising, and mentoring residents free of cost when my White counterparts receive payments for these tasks. I want to see intersectionality inform how we think about problems, sameness, difference, and power. Ezra does too, and he shows us in his chapter on psychiatric disability how people with mental disorders need services that facilitate their recovery. Helping a soccer teammate with language impairments sensitized Ezra to the power of empathy and the ability to change the rules of the game when we contemplate adaptations for people who belong to historically disadvantaged groups. That lesson served as an impetus for him to redesign services that emphasized patient priorities—food, housing, employment, and social connections—when he was a senior administrator at a community mental health center.

Toward these ends, we should think deeply about the range of questions that Ezra asks at the end of each chapter to view ourselves in terms of not just race but also the multitude of characteristics that inform our identities. To incorporate intersubjectivity and intersectionality in our work, we should ask how the complicated matrix of our identities shapes *every* interaction with others through differences in power. At the same time, as Ezra once said, race is not the defining feature of identity for every Black person in the United States, so we should be listening to the factors that patients—indeed, all of us—make central to their life stories. Appreciating that power differences exist, even when they may not be readily redressed (as is the case between the psychiatrist and the incarcerated individual), is one way to evolve an ethics based on the dignity of all human lives that Ezra spotlights.

*Neil Krishan Aggarwal, M.D., M.A.*
*Professor of Clinical Psychiatry, Columbia University*
*Research Psychiatrist, New York State Psychiatric Institute*

# References

Aggarwal NK: Intersubjectivity, transference, and the cultural third. Contemp Psychoanal 47(2):204–223, 2011

Aggarwal NK: The evolving culture concept in psychiatric cultural formulation: implications for anthropological theory and psychiatric practice. Cult Med Psychiatry 47(2):555–575, 2023

Aggarwal NK: The Cultural Formulation Interview in case formulations: a state-of-the-science review. Behav Ther 55(6):1130–1143, 2024 39443057

American Psychiatric Association: Diagnostic and Statistical Manual of Mental Disorders, 4th Edition. Washington, DC, American Psychiatric Association, 1994

American Psychiatric Association: Diagnostic and Statistical Manual of Mental Disorders, 5th Edition. Washington, DC, American Psychiatric Association, 2013

Cho S, Crenshaw KW, McCall L: Toward a field of intersectionality studies: theory, applications, and praxis. Signs (Chic) 38(4):785–810, 2013

Duvivier RJ, Buckley PF, Martin A, et al: International medical graduates in the United States psychiatry workforce. Acad Psychiatry 46(4):428–434, 2022

Good BJ, Fischer MMJ, Willen SS, et al (eds): A Reader in Medical Anthropology: Theoretical Trajectories, Emergent Realities. West Sussex, UK, Wiley-Blackwell, 2010

Griffith E: Forensic psychiatrists and cultural connectedness. J Forensic Psychiatry 7(3):477–479, 1996

Griffith EE: Ethics in forensic psychiatry: a cultural response to Stone and Appelbaum. J Am Acad Psychiatry Law 26(2):171–184, 1998

Griffith EEH, Baranoski MV: Commentary: the place of performative writing in forensic psychiatry. J Am Acad Psychiatry Law 35(1):27–31, 2007

Griffith EEH, Baranoski M: Oral performance, identity, and representation in forensic psychiatry. J Am Acad Psychiatry Law 39(3):352–363, 2011

Gupta A, Ferguson J: Beyond "culture": space, identity, and the politics of difference. Cult Anthropol 7(1):6–23, 1992

Hemmings CP: Rethinking medical anthropology: how anthropology is failing medicine. Anthropol Med 12(2):91–103, 2005

Jordan A, Shim RS, Rodriguez CI, et al: Psychiatry diversity leadership in academic medicine: guidelines for success. Am J Psychiatry 178(3):224–228, 2021

Kirmayer LJ: Cultural psychiatry in historical perspective, in Textbook of Cultural Psychiatry. Edited by Bhugra D, Bhui K. Cambridge, UK, Cambridge University Press, 2007, pp 3–19

Lawrence-Lightfoot S, Davis JH: The Art and Science of Portraiture. San Francisco, CA, Jossey-Bass, 1997

Littlewood R: Psychiatry's culture. Int J Soc Psychiatry 42(4):245–268, 1996 9023608

Lock M: The tempering of medical anthropology: troubling natural categories. Med Anthropol Q 15(4):478–492, 2001

Mezzich JE, Kirmayer LJ, Kleinman A, et al: The place of culture in DSM-IV. J Nerv Ment Dis 187(8):457–464, 1999

Pierce CM: Ezra E. H. Griffith, M.D.: President, American Orthopsychiatric Association, 1997–1998. Am J Orthopsychiatry 67(3):338–340, 1997

Reitz AK, Motti-Stefanidi F, Asendorpf JB: Mastering developmental transitions in immigrant adolescents: the longitudinal interplay of family functioning, developmental and acculturative tasks. Dev Psychol 50(3):754–765, 2014

Useem RH, Downie RD: Third-culture kids. Today's Education 65(3):103–105, 1976

# Introduction
## On the Making of This Text

This book describes my wanderings as a cultural psychiatrist over a 5-year period between 2019 and 2024. My path is sometimes direct and purposeful. At other times, I just meander; or I sit still in contemplation. I focus on people, the places and spaces they occupy, and their well-being or general health. The latter includes, as should be expected, my interest in people's psychological health but not in a neuroscientific fashion. My background and clinical training tend to lead me toward considering individuals' psychosocial experiences. This is a way of integrating the psychological and social dimensions of mundane living. I use brief narratives, short stories, to communicate with my audience and illustrate what I have learned from my observations and experiences. I invite readers on my journeys from the United States to places like Barbados, Great Britain, France, Scotland, Italy, the Czech Republic, and Morocco. The people I met came from those countries, as well as from Nigeria, South Africa, Spain, Algeria, Trinidad, and Russia. My observations are also informed by academic literature and the writings that appear in major daily and monthly periodicals.

## Background

In early 2019, I was invited to write a column for *Psychiatric News*, the now-monthly organ of the American Psychiatric Association. The periodical caters to a readership of thousands of psychiatrists, other mental health professionals, and individuals from related disciplines in the United States and abroad. Its focused interest is on the complex foundation of biomedical sciences, politics, law, public policy, social sciences, and humanities that contribute to the understanding of psychiatric illnesses. This knowledge base in turn undergirds the provision of clinical services that help maintain the well-being of individuals who endure these disorders.

As expected, I set about contemplating how to use my allocated space. I noted that *Psychiatric News* already covered the traditional areas of biomedical psychiatry (including research, scholarship, and clinical pedagogy), legislative and political matters, and patient advocacy. I then considered my interests, which have been developed and sharpened over many years at Yale University, where I served as professor of psychiatry and of African American studies for 20 years. Thus, it was natural for me to turn to the psychosocial arena, where I could make good use of my attraction to narrative, cultural studies, biographical studies, race matters, and questions of colonization that are constantly on my mind. The joint appointments, in a faculty of medicine and a faculty of arts and sciences, provided me with special vantage points from which to explore subjects that have long been tied together in my theorizing and reflection.

I could comfortably write about inequity and justice, ethics-based behavior in medicine, and the extreme environments in which African Americans and other minorities often find themselves. Many of us agree that elements such as poverty, repeated discrimination, poor education, chronic serious illness, and incarceration influence the type of health and mental health that people experience. My strong roots in psychiatry and African American studies played a part in my turn to narrative and biography, as well as my explorations of the Black church. I settled on the title for my monthly column and completed, between 2019 and 2024, more than 60 columns in the "On Mental Health, People, and Places" department. I wanted my writing to provoke reflection, inquiry, and debate about what I might distill for the record of my movements.

## Change in the Air

I emphasize here that many other scholars and I began to notice a transformation taking place in the United States as the 21st century settled down. A peculiar discontent and fear permeated the culture. Yale University Professor Hazel Carby (2021) talked of the "material and symbolic anxieties of the present" that perhaps began around 2016 with Donald Trump's ascension to the presidency of the United States. Then, "a sense of emergency, of imminent threat" became palpable (Carby 2021). Carby referred to the following 4 years of Trump's presidency as at least contributing to the increase in authoritarianism and the spread of white supremacist hatred and violence that so characterized these times. I suspect that Black people and other minority groups were especially attuned to this racialized tinge showing up on everything. The development in American psychiatry was evident, too, with several scholars interrogating the field about its commitment to a more socially oriented form of psychoanalysis. This was in addition to a renewed intellectual interest in the psychologically pernicious effects of racism. Several colleagues and I (Griffith et al. 2023) described this increasing sociocultural and ethnocultural consciousness in psychiatric practice and commentary.

I gradually came to see these new themes in the academy and the broader social world as plaited with other strands of malady, such as climate change, economic hardship, and the raucous presence of the coronavirus disease 2019 (COVID-19). Even leisure activities took a back seat to the upheaval. In times gone by, for example, sacred institutional cows existed, like schools and churches. I do not remember, growing up, that church members anywhere would talk openly of needing to carry guns during a church service to deter attacks from outsiders. In my medical training, I had learned about viruses. But the 1918 influenza fury was only a historical footnote in public health classes for my generation. Even my military service in Vietnam was now visible only in my rearview mirror. Friends of mine, born in the 1940s, loved talking about looking forward to retirement and contemplating trivia concerning the best soccer player in the last 50 years or what was the latest best film or book. Now, the sociopolitical world seems so different.

## Envisioning the Book

As I took in the developments I just discussed, I slowly formulated the plan to incorporate the columns into a book. I decided to make more structured observations about people, their places or spaces, and their fundamental wishes for good health and well-being. I embraced the idea that my writing would be influenced by my years as a Black man whose upbringing was spent in colonial Barbados and New York's Brooklyn, an undergraduate education at Harvard University, and medical studies at the University of Strasbourg in France. I also had an unforgettable year of military service in Vietnam followed by almost 40 years of scholarly life at Yale University.

I contemplated themes for the column series, and because of the obvious limitation of space, I settled on the idea that each essay would constitute a relatively brief narrative of a unique experience. I would focus on individuals I encountered in some distinctive place in the present or the past. An early column topic, "Visibility in a Psychiatric Hospital's Museum" (Griffith 2019b), was an excellent example of this, especially because it related so powerfully to mental health and to a unique example of place in the form of a psychiatric sanitarium. Indeed, in the very first column, I celebrated this connection between geography and health. I emphasized the notion of a healing environment, where individuals interact to the benefit of their health with their architectural surroundings. In that instance, I also referred to the work of Eileen Hogan, a British painter who focused on British parks. I reflected on contemporary ideas that individuals whom I did not know had developed in the literature or in the daily execution of their professional roles. A relevant example was the column on "When Diversity Is Not Enough" (Griffith 2019a), in which I complained that the formulaic integration of people is not the same as cultivating respect for them.

I developed short narratives about different cultures: a story about memorializing dignity and identity in Barbadian public monuments (Griffith 2021a) and a psychiatric discussion of diversity and curiosity about the other in American psychiatry (Griffith 2021e). I focused on the discussion of a play setting in Algeria about the use of violence in resisting colonial oppression (Griffith 2021i). I highlighted our reactions to experiences and events in our lives, with COVID-19 as context (Griffith 2021c). The background was, of course, the cultural fabric that surrounds us and which we would all like to control more. Powerful forces influence the formation of our backgrounds. Some examples are racialized and class-based political disputes, identity politics that defy easy resolution, and pervasive feelings of individual disenchantment. There is also the persistent search for a sense of human dignity and personal worth and the uncertainty about the future in terms of health and security. The pandemic turned those catalysts upside down and produced extensive dislocation in the general culture but, thankfully, not forever.

The stories in this book come through my pen, and I do my best to preserve the authenticity of my observations and my conversations with others. The promise is important to me, as I have profound respect for the idea of collective humanity. There are no hypotheses to prove or disprove, no intention to demonstrate that the individuals in this text have lived rightly or wrongly. I bear witness to acts of

# Introduction

living life in communities in particular eras. The text is a qualitative, culture-based collection of narratives. I leave it to readers to judge the struggles and techniques that people employ in their daily lives. This is the kind of thoughtfulness and debate I wish to evoke. I discussed the patients of the Sainte-Anne Psychiatric Hospital in Paris (Griffith 2019b) and the ones in rehabilitation at the outpatient clinic in New Haven, Connecticut (Griffith 2021b). I illustrated how they used art to establish who they were and wanted to become. We wonder what blocked or facilitated their dreams.

In another column, Louis Menand expressed personal ideas of freedom and the elements that might influence different aspects of public policy (Griffith 2021f). I took pleasure in recounting what a flamenco guitarist (Griffith 2021h), a classical pianist (Griffith 2022b), and steel pan players (Griffith 2020a) communicated in their music. I contemplated the different ways people used sacred spaces: a Russian concert of choral music performed in the church of a Paris neighborhood (Griffith 2022a), an art exhibition in an urban church in London with available coffee for the weary (Griffith 2022c), and pastoral care being offered to gay parishioners in Edinburgh (Griffith 2021g). Using sacred spaces in differentiated relationships with God is so marvelously intriguing and linked to dissimilar views of community and customs. And what to say about the leaders' conceptualizations of their institutions and about regrets in the lives they have lived? Were they pleased with the secular administrative decisions related to the spiritual mission? What did they use to guide their decisions about a moral life? These ideas all deserve contemplation. However, the reader must slow down and assimilate these microlandscapes of mundane activity to link the external interactions with people's inner lives. The resulting information leads to a clearer view of people's well-being.

I turn now to examine three elements—race matters, place, and narrative—that have special status in the text. These themes are also guideposts that help in the understanding of the book's conceptual organization.

## Race Matters

As I matured in my academic life at Yale, I took more careful notice of events around me. I grew more curious about the people I met along the way in work or leisure settings. I remained in close touch with the buddies who were companions during those early years in my old Barbadian village. By the 21st century, race problems in the United States certainly seemed more palpable. It was easy to be aware of the scholarly attention being given to such subjects. My own text, *Belonging, Therapeutic Landscapes, and Networks* (Griffith 2018), saw print during this confusion, as literature about increasing compassion and empathy in psychiatry appeared on the upswing.

Later, there appeared this determined reconstruction of race relations in many institutions, melded with new discussions of what caste, diversity, equity, and inclusion meant. Even the American Psychiatric Association, my main professional group, began holding meetings to contemplate structural racism in its midst. Everybody was aglow with the novel truth that it was unjust to mock others based on ethnicity, skin color, and social standing. My columns "The Knee on the Other's Neck" (Griffith 2021d) and "On Caste and Suffering" (Griffith 2020b) capture this era of reminiscing about the injustice and violence of racial discrimination. The search for reconciliation still seems so elusive, and the compulsive quest for dignity continues because inequity remains acceptable in some quarters.

Readers will remark on my considerable emphasis on dignity throughout the book and the focus of the chapter on "Pursuing Dignity." With the brevity of the columns, I invite readers to sit quietly and consider where they locate themselves in this uneasy discussion of race matters. In this chapter, I often take a novel, crisp narrative approach to the topic. The burden is on readers to find their positions relative to the story and where, after reflection, they want to be positioned. It is an important experience and, ultimately, a lesson to take away. Furthermore, I want readers to appreciate that race matters are not the only elements operative in people's multistoried lives. Neither is racism the only significant form of discrimination.

# Centrality of Place

It turned out that for several months in 2019, I was in France and, for a short time, in England. I was reminded at the time that the exchange between me and foreign cultures favors my sense of intellectual freedom and leads to a clearer understanding of the stimuli I experience within the culture. I understood that there would be a resulting connection between geographic place and the effect on my columns' content. I discussed this notion elsewhere, stating that places provide meaning for us all. For some, it includes a sense of identity, security, family life, and employment. Other times, place signifies maltreatment and indignity. In several of my first few columns, I concentrated on landscapes in Europe, especially France, where I studied medicine and became more familiar with its ties to colonialism in North Africa and West Africa. Similarly, readers will appreciate that throughout the 5 years of columns, Barbados reemerges from time to time, instructing me in the finer art of seeking independence of spirit and body. It is in Barbados, too, that I first encountered the effects of COVID-19. I was on the island for an extended stay when in early 2020, the Anglican Church issued new public health guidelines on how to celebrate the Holy Eucharist. Within a few weeks, all the churches were suddenly closed, the result of this fierce blizzard from COVID-19. The effect was evident on how we wrote, thought, spoke, and interacted with neighbors. Meanwhile, the United States, as home space, sharpened my observations and insights about the racialized psychiatric thinking required as I engaged with notions of caste and discrimination.

Readers will find *place* to be an intrusively ubiquitous element throughout the book. It is melded with racialized thinking, linked to discussions of violence, and an unavoidable presence in any talk of culture. Place corrupts memory at times, makes memory joyful, and enhances the recollection of a musical concert. Some people don't care where they eat. I still see my concentration on a hot dog as I strolled along eating it on the Champs Élysées in Paris one Sunday morning after church. Another intrusive example of place's centrality remains the sound of falling pebbles and dirt on my mother's casket as the cemetery employees filled in her grave. Place reifies cultural happenings, makes geography and events come to life, and serves time as a wonderful companion. It is a crucial element in some of my columns, much like photography. In a variety of the columns, the construct of place appears without my clearly stating it. Still, a certain lesson must be grasped. We are intrinsically linked to where we live, spend leisure time, work, worship, and carry out other meaningful activities.

## Biography and Narrative

I have written about biography and narrative for at least the past two decades. I first published *Race and Excellence* (Griffith 1998) and described an extended dialogue with a mentor, Harvard Professor Chester Pierce. Following that, I wrote the family memoir, *I'm Your Father, Boy* (Griffith 2005), that was set in Barbados. It delved into

Barbadian culture that was powerfully influenced by colonial connections to Britain. *Ye Shall Dream* (Griffith 2010) was focused on the life of a deeply religious modern prophet who founded, in 1957, a faith group that was new to Barbados. The book that I am introducing here is conceptually apart from my earlier work. The new text contrasts appreciably with my previous work in terms of both structure and content. It extends the boundaries of my thinking about narrative. It encompasses more than a single life, more than one unique culture and theme, and it relies on a more purposeful mixture of biography and storytelling. Finally, this collection of columns covers a variety of themes, and the columns are structurally briefer in design.

These forms of narrative scholarship evolved from courses I taught in the Department of African American Studies at Yale University. One course focused on studies of Black autobiographies from different social, professional, and psychological perspectives. Students and I discussed slave narratives and stories from pastors, politicians, musicians, dancers, actors, and so on. The second course addressed biographical storytelling by Caribbean authors. I mixed the themes I cultivated in those two sets of curricula with principles and attitudes acquired in the practice of social and community psychiatry. In addition, I borrowed heavily from anthropological discourse in developing my approach to narrative used in psychiatry and forensic psychiatry.

## Audience and Structure

In this book, I lead psychiatrists and other clinicians to see patients embedded in their social worlds, buffeted by strains and stresses produced by interactions with other people and the sociocultural factors that influence health and well-being. I illustrate how permeable the boundary is between our inner worlds and what surrounds us, that steady maelstrom constantly buffeted by our interactions with culture and other elements I have already mentioned. Other texts traditionally approach this confrontation with social elements through complex and discursive prose. I use experiential, brief narratives to address race matters, explore the concept of place, and raise questions about dignity. I highlight, too, how important it is to recognize that many of us spend considerable time, effort, and energy pursuing personal dignity in various activities. My narrative approach also underlines the beauty in the external world, without flaunting cynicism unduly. By its structure alone, the new text should also appeal to a wide general audience.

# Introduction

In addition to clinician-readers, I want to speak to those who are interested in the anatomy and dynamics of life stories presented in a brief format. This facilitates focus on individualized aspects of a single life. There is also an appeal here to those interested in cultural and African American studies and themes of inequality, social justice, and current affairs.

With the permission of the American Psychiatric Association, I have taken columns that were previously published in *Psychiatric News* between 2019 and 2024 and have edited and reframed them into the next seven chapters of this book. At the beginning of each chapter, the reader will find a section labeled "Columns From *Psychiatric News*" where the previously published columns are grouped. They generally reflect the principal theme of that chapter. For example, in the chapter titled "Considering Race Matters," the columns are based on their connection to themes of race and discrimination. For the next three chapters, their titles are respectively "Pursuing Dignity," "Facing Disability," and "Confronting the COVID-19 Pandemic." I apply consecutively to the next three chapters the following titles: "Talking About Sacred Spaces," "Focusing on Place," and "Seeking Freedom Through the Arts."

In picking up any new text, a reader naturally wonders what in the book's structure is novel and arresting. I use techniques of biography, photography, and medical anthropology to provide insights into theorizing about current themes in the social world. I restate that the columns are purposefully not long. Yet, they demand effort and concentration, a commitment to an adventure of reading about subjects that preoccupy wide swaths of our society, even though they may unfold in unfamiliar and unusual places. It is in their diversity that their richness emerges. There is, too, the privilege of seeing how these individuals have faced significant events in their lives and how they confronted their losses and struggled to regain equilibrium and soldier on in different ways. I have borrowed language from Shoshana Felman and Dori Laub (1992) in their popular text *Testimony* to describe how the stories that I narrate cover a variety of subjects and areas of concern that involve different disciplines and art forms.

Stories always have the potential to serve as models for contemplation of reactions to turmoil and dislocation. They also serve well as a culture-based way of framing the contours of future sociopolitical developments. I emphasize once more my interest in the social world in which we live. I ask readers, through my narratives, to stop, observe, and ponder the description of a microevent: a musical concert, a magazine article, a museum exposition in a foreign country. Readers witness both the written experiences of others and the efforts to try out whether the accounts make sense in the readers' imagined spaces. Readers think about their own lives and whether the stories usefully fit them or are just temporary fantastical flights away from their realities. If the readers engage fully in the voyages, they will find it additionally intriguing to explore the experience through several questions placed at the end of each chapter. In this way, the reader concretizes the academic dimension, comes away confident about what has been learned, and envisions the relevance to clinical work.

# References

Carby HV: The limits of caste. London Review of Books 43(2), January 21, 2021

Felman S, Laub D: Testimony: Crises of Witnessing in Literature, Psychoanalysis, and History. New York, Routledge, 1992

Griffith EEH: Race and Excellence: My Dialogue With Chester Pierce. Iowa City, University of Iowa Press, 1998 (Reprinted by American Psychiatric Association Publishing, 2023)

Griffith EEH: I'm Your Father, Boy: A Family Memoir of Barbados. Tucson, AZ, Hats Off Books, 2005

Griffith EEH: Ye Shall Dream: Patriarch Granville Williams and the Barbados Spiritual Baptists. Kingston, Jamaica, University of the West Indies Press, 2010

Griffith EEH: Belonging, Therapeutic Landscapes, and Networks: Implications for Mental Health Practice. New York, Routledge, 2018

Griffith EEH: When diversity is not enough. Psychiatric News, August 16, 2019a

Griffith EEH: Visibility in a psychiatric hospital's museum. Psychiatric News, December 31, 2019b

Griffith EEH: The steel pan and decolonizing mental health. Psychiatric News, September 24, 2020a

Griffith EEH: On caste and suffering. Psychiatric News, November 16, 2020b

Griffith EEH: Memorializing dignity and identity in public monuments. Psychiatric News, January 1, 2021a

Griffith EEH: Creative writing and psychiatric rehabilitation. Psychiatric News, April 1, 2021b

Griffith EEH: Angels and the pandemic. Psychiatric News, April 30, 2021c

Griffith EEH: The knee on the other's neck. Psychiatric News, May 20, 2021d

Griffith EEH: Diversity and curiosity about the other. Psychiatric News, July 25, 2021e

Griffith EEH: Talking about freedom with Louis Menand. Psychiatric News, July 26, 2021f

Griffith EEH: Peace cranes in a sanctuary. Psychiatric News, October 25, 2021g

Griffith EEH: A flamenco tale in Edinburgh: recreating home. Psychiatric News, November 30, 2021h

Griffith EEH: Yonder on the other side. Psychiatric News, December 29, 2021i

Griffith EEH: On difference and othering. Psychiatric News, February 28, 2022a

Griffith EEH: The solitude of an artist. Psychiatric News, November 30, 2022b

Griffith EEH: The pleasure of chance encounters. Psychiatric News, December 28, 2022c

Griffith EEH, Sreenivasan S, DiCiro MS, et al. Illuminating sociocultural and ethnocultural consciousness in forensic practice. J Am Acad Psychiatry Law 51(2):263–271, 2023

# Considering Race Matters

# Columns From *Psychiatric News*

## When Diversity Is Not Enough[1]

At the American Psychiatric Association's (APA's) Annual Meeting in 2019, it was to the credit of the organization that many sessions focused on matters related to Blacks and other minorities within APA. There were academic discussions that highlighted the historical differences between the APA of decades ago and the present status of the organization. The minority caucuses at this meeting were vibrant, their members active, and the sense of community was palpable. I quietly noted, however, that while advocates of diversity in other organizations have been speaking out and working toward inclusion of minorities, Blacks have not consistently been the beneficiaries of the sustained drumbeating. Other groups seeking fairness and equity in society also deservedly attract attention with their complaints and their demands; however, in American society, many Blacks continue to be caught up in mundane experiences that are persistently racialized. For them, there is this feeling that America is not yet in a postracial phase. This concern is not limited to Blacks and their racial struggle. A casual perusal of the daily lay press suggests that other minority groups are often worried about the enduring nature of their struggles.

After the Annual Meeting, I began rereading *African American Bioethics: Culture, Race, and Identity* (Prograis and Pellegrino 2007). In the book's introduction, Edmund Pellegrino noted that Blacks in the United States commonly face color discrimination and a continuing, personal depreciation by the dominant group. He theorized that these experiences often result in Blacks developing a similar way of thinking about some things and differentiated views on others. The result may well be that Blacks weigh some of their experiences differently from the way in which the dominant group might consider the same events. Pellegrino pointed out that this process could lead to distinctions between the ethics norms of Whites and Blacks.

I was aware of this difference between Blacks and the dominant group some years ago when APA members were discussing outpatient commitment. I argued that we physicians should narrow the use of

---

[1] Adapted with permission from Griffith EEH: On Mental Health, People, and Places: When Diversity Is Not Enough. *Psychiatric News*, August 2019. Copyright © 2019 American Psychiatric Association. All rights reserved.

outpatient commitment because of how it affects the patient's liberty in a community setting. Some members of the dominant group argued for a more liberal stance on use of the intervention. I always believed that my experience with racial discrimination influenced my conservative view of an intervention that is more likely to impinge on Black patients' rights and privileges as citizens.

As I reflected anew on my views, I understood more clearly Pellegrino's idea that in bioethics, it is important to determine how much weight any group's historical experiences and traditions deserve. He did not argue that any one group should carry the day in these conversations. He did suggest, however, that different groups might find common ground in raising concerns about cultural principles that diminish "human flourishing"—a concept of general well-being that has been defined by some scholars as covering domains such as life satisfaction, meaning and purpose, and close social relationships. Pellegrino therefore offered us hope if the groups work together. In retrospect, the 2019 Annual Meeting was a cause for rejoicing. My good friend and colleague Chester Pierce would have been pleased that diversity and inclusion had taken on such meaning. Minority groups were in full voice. Blacks had presence at many different levels in the organization. They were talking about recently published texts focused on Black mental health. Everybody also knew that the president of the organization was a Black woman, and another Black female psychiatrist was poised to become the leader of the American Medical Association.

However, Pellegrino's point was ringing in my ears. Dominant and nondominant groups could well think about moral behavior as a function of their own histories and traditions. Thus, they could view quite differently the effects of psychiatric illness and treatments, depending on whether they had had to struggle with accompanying poverty and racial discrimination. Understanding the effects of involvement with the law enforcement system could further complicate their views. Because of this complexity, it seems obvious that, rejoice all we want, diversity and inclusion are not enough. They are important and necessary but not enough to eliminate all the differences between and among members of a large organization.

If we are to maintain our remarkably impressive gains within this revitalized APA, we must continue working collectively for all members in what I like to call a "genuinely therapeutic space." We must reinforce principles borrowed from Nicholas Christakis's recent text *Blueprint: The Evolutionary Origins of a Good Society* (2019). These principles make up what he calls "The Social Suite," which is characterized by commitment to individual identity; affection for partners, friendship, and social networks; affinity for our own group not linked to rejection of others; appreciation of the goodness in others; and cooperation. Of course, sustained excellence in leadership is always helpful, especially when it embodies a recognition of everyone's inherent self-worth.

## Black Identity Politics and Psychiatry[2]

The sequestration caused by the present pandemic has produced for me at least one beneficent outcome: The time to reread and ponder articles published some time ago. I returned recently to a piece by Harvard Professor Orlando Patterson (2006) titled "Being and Blackness." In it, Patterson comments on two books. However, my interest here centers only on Tommie Shelby's *We Who Are Dark: The Philosophical Foundations of Black Solidarity* (2007).

Patterson (2006) makes clear from the start that Shelby dismisses "the notion of an inherent or essential Black identity, the idea that one shares some deep-seated common bond or kinship with all black people by virtue of being black." Shelby disposes, too, of the idea that "being black means one is, or ought to be, culturally black." In contrast, Patterson states that Shelby promotes a form of pragmatic nationalism that advocates Black solidarity, despite the racial composition of the political organization in which Blacks and Whites may be operating. Patterson claims that Shelby's Black solidarity is characterized by "special concern, loyalty, and trust" that is distinct from notions of a color-blind liberal reform effort. This Black solidarity is related to Blacks' history of slavery and race-based discrimination.

I had to be attentive in reading this analysis, as Patterson notes that Black solidarity in this form may not be the solution in every context. For example, Blacks must understand that the socioeconomic challenge they will confront in the United States may not always be linked to their Blackness. Still, Shelby seems to grant that Blacks legitimately have "shared political interests" related to their "racial subordination and their collective resolve to triumph over it."

---

[2] Adapted with permission from Griffith EEH: On Mental Health, People, and Places: Black Identity Politics and Psychiatry. *Psychiatric News*, August 2020. Copyright © 2020 American Psychiatric Association. All rights reserved.

I confess there is a certain laziness in making excursions into philosophical territory through the eyes of another scholar. However, in this case I felt the trip worthwhile, as it provided a different view of the current context surrounding the struggle over Blacks' rights and privileges in modern America. Tommie Shelby's work also clarified for me the new eruptions of Black-White discord within the APA. Yes, Black members of APA are palpably upset about their perceived treatment within the Association, and the present national climate reinforces their irritation.

There is little point in fanning the flames of discord here in a brief commentary. Still, I have talked with APA members on different sides of the debate and have reached the conclusion that the organization's leadership has more work to do in structuring the discourse. Some of this further effort will require clearer avoidance of rigid boundaries and arguments that emphasize power and legalistic positions. I acknowledge the important step taken by our president, Dr. Jeffrey Geller, in establishing the Task Force to Address Structural Racism Throughout Psychiatry. I have hopes for its advancement of conversations among our diverse constituencies and emphasis on mutual and attentive listening.

This is 2020, not 1969 when Black members of APA were obliged to raise their voices with strident belligerence. Blacks want seats at the influential tables of APA, and Whites must understand that Blacks are tired of repeated begging. Such behavior is below the new standard of dignity for minority group members. Blacks must in turn appreciate that they are not the only nondominant group in the organization or the broader society. Thus, making what Shelby (2007) calls "chauvinistic claims" about Black people's heritage and privileges is often problematic when pursuing political action.

There is also no denying APA's economic and political reach in the marketplace. These bilateral acknowledgments affirm that Blacks and Whites are inextricably intertwined in this organization. There is no going back on this point, and all APA constituencies must recognize this reality. I am confident that Jeffrey Geller wants to build community in the organization. I expect he appreciates that every action toward this end must result in mutual preservation of the other's dignity. However, in closing, I return to Orlando Patterson's reference to being and Blackness. The entire constellation of APA's leadership will benefit from conversations, guided by colleagues with experience in the trauma of racism, about those of us who are dark.

# Hate in the Context of Oppression[3]

In an earlier column, I noted that the coronavirus disease 2019 (COVID-19) pandemic stimulated my reflecting on articles published some time ago. Here, I discuss a piece sent by a friend who has a deep interest in solving problems evoked by oppression and discrimination. The article, "Surviving Hating and Being Hated: Some Personal Thoughts About Racism From a Psychoanalytic Perspective," was written by the psychoanalyst Kathleen Pogue White (2002) and published in *Contemporary Psychoanalysis*.

Dr. White invites the reader to ponder racial hatred. She does not define it crisply. However, the clinical vignettes she provides evoke intense animosity or hostility. She calls hatred a common human experience, one that we fear and that forces us into a collusion of silence. It is understood that, while her focus is on the racial context, people experience hatred and hating on other bases like gender, religion, language, and disability. She exhorts us to tear the veil off this taboo, get it out in the open. Let fresh air into the space. Our clinical work might improve. I suggest that so may our social interactions and political discourse.

She sees three ways of thinking about racial hatred: being hated, hating the self, and hating the other. She emphasizes that her model derives from her experiences. For the first concept, she tells us about her kindergarten interaction with a nun. The nun asked whether anyone could read. Young Kathleen put her hand up to announce her achievement in reading. The nun replied that her pupil was not telling the truth. Dr. White goes through some psychoanalytic commentary before concluding that the nun spat poison on a youngster. The hatred continued as the teacher persisted in calling her some sort of rotten fruit throughout grade school. The analyst-author explains that there is a strategy for surviving this hatred: recognizing the projection from the nun, getting angry, and turning it back. So much for the problem of being hated.

White employs similar brief stories in talking about hating the self, which she defines as the internalization of negative attributes and projections. Her explication of these processes is important. She wants to

---

[3] Adapted with permission from Griffith EEH: On Mental Health, People, and Places: Hate in the Context of Oppression. *Psychiatric News*, September 2020. Copyright © 2020 American Psychiatric Association. All rights reserved.

assure us that the psychoanalytic method may offer a pathway to healing. I reminded myself that there must be a role for positive experiences coming from others around us: at home, work, and leisure, for example.

White's third way of thinking about hatred has to do with hating the other. This response is variable, as we all know. It may take the form of a quiet rebuke, a serene sit-in, a rambunctious march, or a frightening manifestation of plundering and violence. She calmly wonders what internal pressures on Whites colonizing America may have caused them to hate Blacks and other groups, with resulting revulsion and outright murder. She suggests the mayhem of those early colonizing years may have been produced by the toxicity involved in the colonizers' expulsion from their original countries. She invites White people to mull this problem over, as she lays bare her own pronounced hatred toward them.

Kathleen White leaves the meaty challenges for last. She notes,

> For blacks to come out of collusive racial self-hatred, we have to take back the good projections (white is good) and tolerate the experience of our own self-hatred (black is bad). For whites to break the collusion of racial hating, they have to take back the bad projections (black is bad) and tolerate the experience of whatever self-hatred they experience as a result. (White 2002, p. 421)

These recommendations are complicated by our traditions and habits, White points out. We are accustomed to reflecting on what it means to be Black. Now, how about considering the experience of being White?

Other scholars have been recognizing this new turn in our field, leading to a renewed exploration of "White privilege." My late colleague Professor Frederick Hickling (2009) had for some years been using the term *European-American psychosis*. He raised questions about the birth of this delusional idea that Whites are inherently superior to everybody else. In her Fanon-esque psychoanalytic model, White points out that both the oppressor and the oppressed are caught up in a collusion related to racial hatred. Unraveling it requires a joint agreement to self-examine (see Figure 1.1). It is a tough assignment, as we are inclined to attack the blameworthy other. White wants more than that, although she concedes she may not see it in her lifetime. She urges us to end the bilateral self-hating legacy of racism. The crucial first step is for us to talk about it.

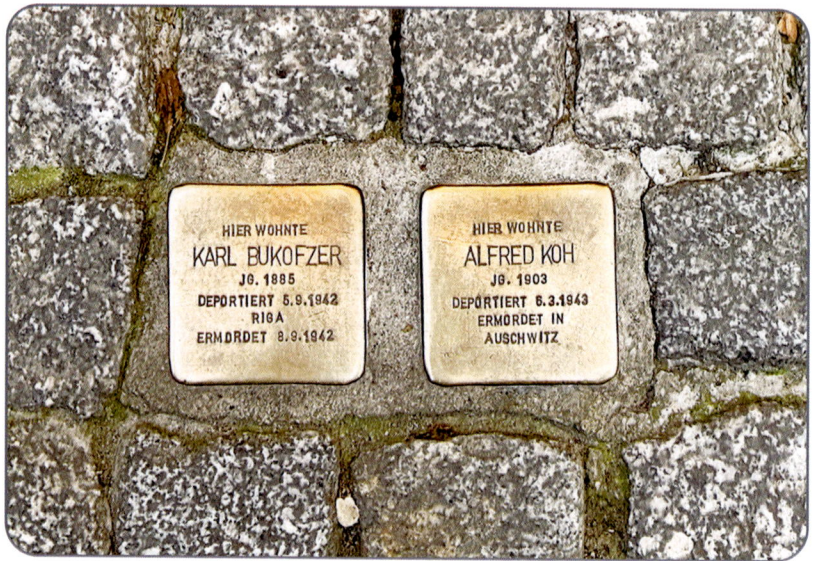

**Figure 1.1** An Exemplar of *Stolpersteine* in Berlin, Germany.

These "stumbling stones" are decentralized monuments to the hatred and oppression of the Holocaust and are ubiquitous. They display a victim's name, birthdate, date of deportation, and concentration camp.

*Source.* Photograph by Brigitte Griffith.

## On Caste and Suffering[4]

In her new book, *Caste: The Origins of Our Discontents*, Isabel Wilkerson (2020, p. 25) said it plainly: "A caste system has a way of filtering down to every inhabitant, its codes absorbed like mineral springs, setting the expectations of where one fits on the ladder." On several occasions, I have confronted the experience of being presumed to be at the bottom of the ladder. Someone had thought the presumption was justified by what Wilkerson calls an immutable trait. Yes, at every turn the trait was mine, and I could do nothing about it. Wilkerson is right in stating that the categorization process is about the exercise of power by those who see themselves in the presumed superior group.

---

[4] Adapted with permission from Griffith EEH: On Mental Health, People, and Places: On Caste and Suffering. *Psychiatric News*, November 2020. Copyright © 2020 American Psychiatric Association. All rights reserved.

Caste is a major structural and functional problem in many societies. Wilkerson calls it a sort of ranking system that determines one's value and practical status in everyday life transactions. Caste, of course, brings with it suffering. Once a group of people decide that, on the caste scale they have invented, they are above others, they feel the impulse to reify it and lord it over the others. They articulate in different ways what Wilkerson calls the "centrality" of their self-created superiority. Then, they rank others in descending order of closeness to the superior ones. Wilkerson clarifies the rationales and characteristics of these systems. She demonstrates how far some individuals go to maintain the elaborate structures on which hang the ladders of hierarchy.

Over the years, I have noted how commonly we avoid understanding that human suffering, derived from this ranking of human value and usage, is ubiquitous. Many of those at the bottom of the rank ladder argue that their experiences of suffering are intrinsic to their identity. They may also feel that their pain, no matter how it is measured, is more intense than the suffering of others. However, Wilkerson asserts that different forms of caste structure are comparable because of the pervasive intensity of the suffering that the victims must endure. Thus, we should expect that the racist caste system of the United States, the structural problem of caste in India, and systems in other disparate geographies have similar characteristics. Of course, all of them still retain distinctive features. The most important consideration is that we all ultimately understand that caste has the power to become the very heart of systems that operate economic, political, and social interactions. That is the major implication of Wilkerson's theorizing, and I add that the significance for the public health of citizenry should be obvious.

It is useful to contemplate caste in the context of smaller reference frames, such as the inpatient psychiatric service or even the psychiatric hospital. In these more circumscribed spaces, the sociopolitical economy is not grandly evident. Nevertheless, through attentive observation, one can uncover evidence of Michel Foucault's notion of disciplinary power at work in a clinic through a medical caste system (Foucault 1963). The physician-anthropologist Véronique A. S. Griffith (2020) and others point out that this system may operate on sources of power such as sociolegal authority and knowledge exchange. Consequently, young professionals, just out of medical or nursing school, begin to see that they have leadership roles to fill. They have an expertise to flaunt, and they grow progressively into their positions of superiority over the patients who need their care. The caregivers eventually realize that their status, professional socialization, and mundane interactions have prepared them for these assignments of governance.

Caregivers, feeling their organizational strength, may learn how to withhold and dispense privileges. They may label as bad a patient who is unable to conform to social rules and then treat that patient with minimal compassion. Some patients will lose their autonomy, and others will receive less than optimal care. Under the pressure of this medical caste system, it is easy to forget that the patient's position should be rooted in citizen values such as freedom, autonomy, privacy, and equality. I know that in recent decades colleagues have worked hard to weaken this disciplinary power system and to enhance patients' participation in their care and in communication with their caregivers. However, this positive accomplishment seems under threat from the influence of the coronavirus. The virus has caused erosion of patient influence resulting from transformations in the structure of caregiving. We must remember that patients and caregivers are on a collaborative journey, not engaged in a caste enterprise benefiting those at the top of the ladder.

## The Knee on the Other's Neck[5]

> If we—and now I mean the relatively conscious whites and the relatively conscious blacks, who must, like lovers, insist on, or create the consciousness of the others—do not falter in our duty now, we may be able, handful that we are, to end the racial nightmare, ... and change the history of the world.
> 
> —James Baldwin, *The Fire Next Time* (1963)

The recurring visual tableau of Derek Chauvin's knee on the neck of George Floyd is the unavoidable central scene of all stories focused on this historic trial of Mr. Chauvin by the state of Minnesota. A former Minneapolis police officer, Mr. Chauvin was sentenced in April 2021 to 22.5 years in prison for the second-degree murder of George Floyd. Commentary on the jury's verdict will reverberate for a long time. In contemplating my reactions to the Chauvin verdict, I thought it would be helpful to look back at an unusual encounter I had with a police officer some years ago. I wanted a personal point of reference as I continued writing this piece. So, with my memories at hand, I examined several reports about the legal decision. They came to my attention

---

[5] Adapted with permission from Griffith EEH: On Mental Health, People, and Places: The Knee on the Other's Neck. *Psychiatric News*, June 2021. Copyright © 2021 American Psychiatric Association. All rights reserved.

by chance, in unsolicited email messages or through my haphazard perusal of daily news media.

My experience with the police officer might not meet the standards evident in Erik Erikson's discussions of "the event" in Gandhi's life (Erikson 1970). I cannot claim that my encounter constituted a fateful turn in my life course. Or a fork at which I worried about the path I had been forced onto. However, I have mulled over that soundless, fleeting interaction with my officer on numerous occasions. I know its indelibility, its singularity, and its invisibility. There were no cell phones present to record it for the future. I have used the memory in sifting the chaff from the wheat in the discourse surrounding *Chauvin*.

I was driving along a narrow city street on the Yale University campus when I spotted a Black colleague I had not seen in a long time. I parked the car in the open space next to a fire hydrant and invited him to chat. I kept the car running to make it obvious that I could easily move if asked to do so. We were both dressed in jacket and tie and calmly minding our own business in the middle of the day. After a few minutes, a uniformed White police officer approached from behind, on the driver's side. Seeing him, I lowered the window. He gave me a summons for parking there, said nothing, and walked back to his own vehicle. My friend and I simultaneously asked why he had not just ordered us to move or at least said something that recognized his official act. We then considered the option of complaining and decided to avoid any further interaction with this officer. We felt he was unfriendly and seeking some sort of confrontation. Since we were Black and outnumbered him, we thought he might try to escalate things and get us all into an unnecessary struggle. We felt it would be silly to turn the joy of our mini reunion into something we might regret for a long time. We said goodbye to each other, and I drove off.

We have rediscussed this circumstance several times over the passing months, pleased that we returned home safe that day. The officer could justify his actions based on the idea that blocking a fire hydrant is unlawful. He was within his rights to punish us for the infraction without first asking us to move. Nevertheless, we were angry and upset. The officer did not utter a word. The act, done in silence, did not recognize us. He perpetrated an unfriendly deed, and we did not trust him. As Matthew Alemu (2021), a University of Michigan sociologist, explained in a *Detroit Free Press* column, "It's hard to find the words to express how it feels, as a Black male, to have to process these events." Then he talked of being honestly afraid at such moments. The collective fear, my friend's and mine, was palpable. Alemu asked whether our citizenship must be "contingent on our willingness to accept eternal inequality." The context framed all one wants to know about a policeman's power and being treated in an undignified way.

It is a natural first step to hope that proper training of police will improve things. However, those of us interested in these phenomena know that one-sided training exercises are rarely enough. In that case, I turn to other explanatory mechanisms I have discussed elsewhere before. That officer and we needed a sustained interactive experience so we could tell him about our fear of his power and his weapon. He could, in turn, recount his feelings toward Black men who put their cars next to fire hydrants in the middle of the day and chat as though they have no pressing cares. However, in truth, I know nothing about what undergirded his decisions concerning lawbreakers. I never met him again. Perhaps he, too, was afraid.

I have occasionally discussed this incident with White and Black police officers. They said consistently that my friend and I did the wise thing. They advised walking away and celebrating life with our families. I have even questioned them about the cowardice in our defensive behavior. They smiled and said calmly that avoiding conflict with an officer beats a hospital stay and an arrest. Still, none of this gets at understanding why my officer did not at first strike a position of reasonable neutrality and ask me to move the vehicle. The psychoanalyst Anton Hart (2020), writing about what he calls diversity-related pedagogy, advocates cultivation of curiosity about the "other." I presume this invitation mandates taking this stance toward all officers. However, the tableau of the knee on the neck gets in the way. It demands hostility toward the knee's owner and blunts our potential interest in and cultivation of a generous spirit toward those who possess the power to hurt us. When the hurt is aimed at our dignity, our anger can be unforgiving.

There is an important lesson here. The officer in my vignette did not put a Chauvin-type knee on my neck. His act was not so baldly violent. It was, nevertheless, oppressive. It troubled my composure and evoked fear; it lowered my dignity and disrupted my confidence as a productive citizen. My officer's behavior borrows its power from a tradition of pervasive police supremacy. Sometimes it borders on the criminal, as we know well (see Figure 1.2). That is the way it is in many democratic societies, especially where racialized thinking operates. The trouble is that little attention is paid to what the policeman is thinking when he deploys his power. I am also concerned that the sense of supremacy is visible in other systems besides law enforcement. That leads to the

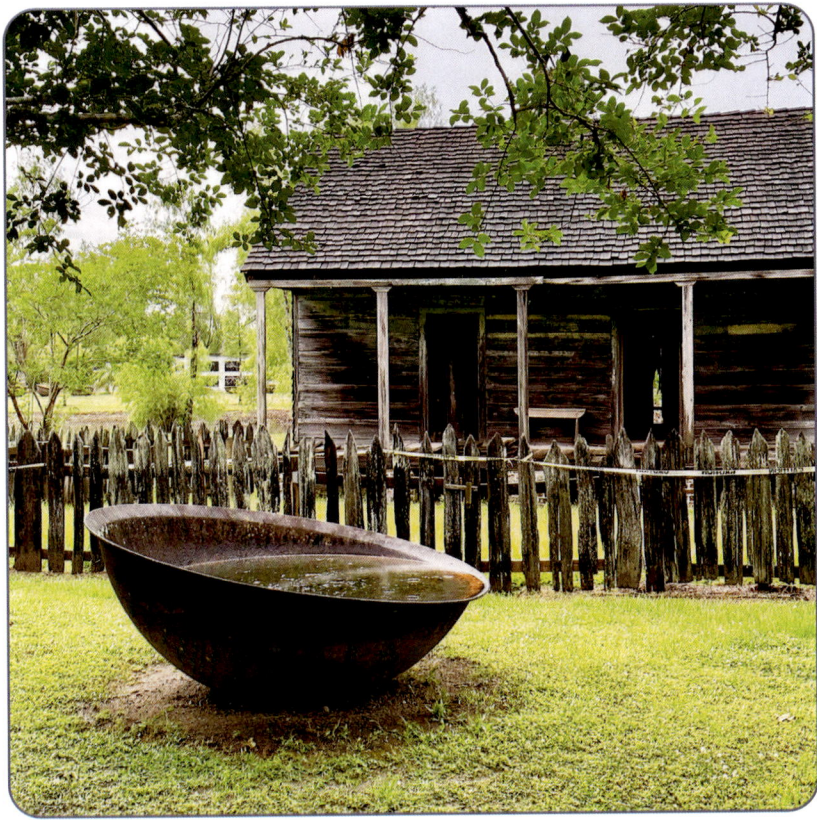

**Figure 1.2** The Whitney Plantation of Louisiana.

Opened in 2014 as a museum dedicated to the history of slavery, it started as an indigo plantation around 1752. The photograph shows a sugar kettle standing in front of a cabin where enslaved people lived.

*Source.*  Photograph by Brigitte Griffith.

unavoidable conclusion that while Derek Chauvin's behavior may be aberrant because of its duration, outcome, and public nature, it should not be considered a rare exemplar of interpersonal violence. I admit, too, that my personal experience has encouraged a more empathic curiosity and view of Chauvin. I understand that there are obscure structural factors that confirm the reality of the officer's power and my fear of it and of him.

Yale President Peter Salovey (2021) issued a letter to members of the university community on the evening of April 20, 2021. In the letter titled "Today's Verdict on the Murder of George Floyd," Salovey termed Floyd's death an "indictment of our nation's failure to address anti-Black violence and racism." He demonstrated cogently and passionately in his public missive that he and his cadre of university officers developed a thoughtful response to these race matters. However, he did not explain why the university took so long to enter the fray. I remember delivering a public lecture at Yale Medical School on the subject of "Belonging at Yale" (Griffith 1990). Few others were concerned then about such matters.

I used another presentation around 2006 to recommend steps I thought the leader of the medical school should take to improve the climate of equity and belonging. Afterward, a few full professors chastised me for giving my advice for all to hear. They were not polite in making clear that I had no right to say anything so pointedly to the dean at the time. Talking about knees and necks in an academic institution!

More recently, the university finally became interested in what it meant for minority groups to belong to this academic community and set up a Committee on Diversity, Inclusion, and Belonging. I wonder what elements would have been needed to foment this interest sooner: fiercer political activism, more intensive questioning about the university's intentions, cultural humility? Now that the university leadership is keen on utilizing its human, sociopolitical, and economic resources in the broad struggle for social justice, the potential impact is breathtaking, especially if sustained.

Charles Blow (2021), *The New York Times* columnist, noted that even in celebrating victories like the *Chauvin* verdict, sadness accompanies the joy. He explained that between the discernible poles that mark progress, minorities develop "hostility, resentment, and contempt." Blow sees value in ritualizing the outcome, as such positive results can be "recharging and restorative." Nevertheless, we must not confuse "the war that still rages for the battle in which we were victorious." The crusade must continue, Blow argued, if change is to emerge from the verdict. Blow emphasized keeping one's eyes on the prize, advancing the struggle for human rights.

In the April 21, 2021, issue of *The Harvard Gazette*, Christina Pazzanese (2021), a Harvard staff writer, reported in her interview of Harvard Professor Cornell Brooks about his reactions to the *Chauvin* verdict. Brooks asserted that *Chauvin* "is by no means a congratulatory moment or a moment of commendation for either the judiciary or policing. It is a moment of challenge, and it's a moment of resolve." Brooks saw the need for multiethnic, multiracial, and multisectoral coalitions to "face down" this problem of racism and police violence. The activism must take place at and on different levels simultaneously. There are roles for all of us. He demanded the passage of the George Floyd Justice in Policing Act (HR 7120). He assigned to media the task of defining a justice narrative that must be heard everywhere. Only then will it penetrate the courts.

Brooks also wanted "a sustained presence of protesters and demonstrators in the streets." Hopefully, that movement will attract participation of the business community and politicians. He suggested that "our confidence, our hopefulness, our sense of optimism" can be found in the "commitment and courage of those around us." Once again, passing laws will not bring total satisfaction. Statutes cannot mandate the earnest curiosity that Anton Hart (2020) suggested we display toward each other. Neither can we forcefully implement that intersubjective recognition of the other's inherent dignity. Brooks essentially broadened Charles Blow's program of making things better through a multipronged approach that relies on a coalition of interdisciplinary participation harnessed by deep commitment from authentic citizenship.

George Floyd and his family were the victims of a terrible episode of violence. Nothing can erase that fact. We must bear witness to that reality and hope that its memory will sustain efforts to make things better for all of us who remain. Seeking justice is hard work. It requires us, on encountering injustice, to accept responsibility for finding a role to change things and make progress. The knee-on-the-neck tableau is not a problem merely for the justice system and police officers. We must think about violence in other contexts, such as in faith communities, universities, workplaces, and political systems. Violence resides in the demeaning behavior of those who oversee others and treat them with scant respect. It demands great resilience not to hate the one whose knee is on your neck. Recognizing this demands a level of spiritual humility that unsettles many of us. Still, it is at the core of working together to make change. Standing arrogantly to the side and demanding that my police officer abase himself and take his traffic ticket back will not achieve lasting change. He and I must chat and figure out why we are so estranged one from the other.

# Diversity and Curiosity About the Other[6]

Colleagues have been shepherding me through readings and discussions of psychoanalytic literature. The enterprise has been enjoyable, as the reading topics have been about race and psychoanalysis. We recently reviewed Anton Hart's "Principles of Teaching Issues of Diversity in a Psychoanalytic Context" (2020). He is a training and supervising analyst on the faculty of the William Alanson White Institute.

In the article, Hart presented a collection of principles for discussing diversity from a psychoanalytic perspective. He was aware, however, that his ideas are applicable to other pedagogical contexts. That is why I recommend the piece for reading outside of psychoanalytic circles. He made clear in a footnote that while he intended to focus on the diversity category of race, his principles are useful in discussions of age, gender, socioeconomic status, and other arenas of difference. Hart's theorizing about methods of teaching diversity is timely, considering all the commentary these days about the need for diversity in organizations and systems. Furthermore, conquering fears of those others, the people we do not really know, has become an urgent national preoccupation.

Hart described 12 principles he collected patiently, which he viewed as optional rather than mandatory notions he wanted readers to approach carefully: he meant that teachers should be simultaneously open to being learners, and learners should also teach. He emphasized the importance of experience and process in an interactive method of inquiry about otherness. Fundamental to his novel pedagogical argument about diversity was the cultivation of openness in our conversations with and about those who are different from us. Hart argued that there is bidirectionality in the process of curiosity. Thus, when we ask about others, it is expected that they may want to know about us.

Hart is not a fan of the traditional method of approaching diversity. This popular pedagogical approach provides knowledge that leads to what is commonly termed *competency and literacy*. For example, it may teach about geography and culture. However, Hart wants more than this emphasis on content. In the absence of earnest curiosity, we are left with avoidance of the required openness that facilitates meaningful engagement with people. Thus, studying otherness in the classroom

---

[6] Adapted with permission from Griffith EEH: On Mental Health, People, and Places: Diversity and Curiosity About the Other. *Psychiatric News*, July 2021. Copyright © 2021 American Psychiatric Association. All rights reserved.

may provide knowledge, but it cannot replace the experience and process of cultivating human interaction.

Hart recognized that certain threats accompany curiosity about the other. He described the possibility of having one's sense of self disturbed through this curiosity. He thinks this may be linked to the possibility that what we learn about ourselves and others, as we inquire, may at times be at odds with what we had imagined. He suggested, too, that being the object of curiosity may cause us to feel objectified and implicitly controlled by those posing the questions. The experience may remind us of sensations related to control and dominance.

So, as teachers pose their questions, students may well ask who wants to know and why. We should assume that in these exercises, both teachers and students have the capacity to be malicious. The clinician in Hart recommended that teachers be thoughtful when they invite students to represent their diversity openly. This is important when the students' otherness is connected to subjugation. Hart concluded with the advice that anyone setting out to teach about diversity should adopt a position reflecting traits of thoughtfulness, openness, and humility.

Anton Hart's contribution to the literature on diversity is important. The insights are couched in a psychoanalytic vocabulary that at first may cause readers to proceed hesitantly. Nonetheless, concentration on the practical dimensions of Hart's theorizing puts his principles in clearer perspective. Certainly, his contrast between cultivating curiosity about the other and the retention of a model focused on knowledge and content eventually takes clearer form. From my vantage point, being curious reinforces recognition of the other's inherent and inviolable dignity. Hart effectively connected the experience of curiosity to his notions of listening and speaking thoughtfully.

## Talking About Freedom With Louis Menand[7]

It is not a habit of mine to listen to podcasts. Purely by accident recently, I came across *The New York Times*' "Book Review Podcast" and "The Ezra Klein Show." The hosts conducted separate interviews of Louis Menand, the popular Harvard professor, critic, and staff writer for

---

[7] Adapted with permission from Griffith EEH: On Mental Health, People, and Places: Talking About Freedom With Louis Menand. *Psychiatric News*, August 2021. Copyright © 2021 American Psychiatric Association. All rights reserved.

*The New Yorker.* On each occasion, he discussed his new book, *The Free World: Art and Thought in the Cold War* (Menand 2021). The research for the text and its preparation apparently took him about 10 years. I also reviewed the written transcript of the discussion from "The Ezra Klein Show" titled "The Freeing of the American Mind" and the book review by David Oshinsky (2021).

Menand's book focused on the first 20 years of the Cold War between 1945 and 1965. Ezra Klein noted that in those two postwar decades between the end of World War II and the emergence of the Vietnam conflict, "ideas were born out of interactions between individuals and larger historical forces." Menand was interested in two types of transformation: those coming from ideas of freedom that powered the arts in new directions and the sociocultural and political changes wrought by major historical forces such as civil rights, the women's movement, and decolonization.

Menand noted his special interest in biography and social history. These disciplines led him to consider how the major movements affected the artistic creativity of several important figures, among them James Baldwin, Jackson Pollack, Jean-Paul Sartre, and Susan Sontag. Pollack's experimentation with the "drip paintings" did not evoke pleasant reactions everywhere. Neither did John Cage convince everyone that the "4 minutes and 33 seconds" of purposeful silence in one of his compositions was a new and worthwhile form of music. Evidently, these fresh expressions of artistic freedom were not comprehensively welcomed by consumers. Nevertheless, change was in the air, and some forms had staying power. Baldwin and Sontag were good examples, even though they also had their detractors.

It was understandable that the happenings wrought by Nazi Germany throughout Europe and elsewhere had affected almost everyone's defining search for liberty. In the sociocultural and political spheres, this was evident in the demands of the Black American soldiers returning from Europe and in Sontag's contributions to the women's movement. These developments in the social, cultural, and political spheres have left their mark on us today, as many witnesses have stated in the last months. Nevertheless, Menand and his interviewers articulated differences between the "freedom" of the 1950s and the present. For example, Menand noted that Martin Luther King Jr. used "freedom" frequently without adding "equality," although he is confident that King did believe in equality. In contrast, George Wallace used "freedom" to justify resistance to enforced segregation. Menand clarified that the foundation of the current civil rights movement is equality. This differentiated discourse, as Menand talked about freedom, highlights the complexity of such conversations. Even I never imagined in the decade of the 1960s that conceptualizing freedom would become so complicated in the coming century.

I found it fascinating to contemplate, in personal terms, the reactive quest for freedom in response to historic movements across wide swaths of geography (see Figure 1.3). This was on the platforms of both culture and politics. Concerning culture, I previously mentioned the rise of the steel pan in Caribbean countries (E.E.H. Griffith 2020) as a visibly powerful and indigenous musical instrument. I have also described its use in European classical music as well as its application to the compositions authored by local artists. I have marveled, too, at the insightful commentary proposed by Caribbean theorists like Professors Frederick Hickling and Richard Drayton. I have loved their work concerning sovereign independence and its implications for freedom in many spheres of mundane living.

There is also the matter of how Menand's theorizing applies to my experience in the academic context, to "elite universities," as he refers to them. Menand seems enamored of the improved access of different social classes to our universities. The class of cultural consumers has widened. That is a good thing. It has also led to greater awareness of social injustice and racial inequity. Menand pointed also to universities' drive to be inclusive now, going "to enormous lengths to make students feel welcome and comfortable, regardless of their backgrounds."

I agree that some universities are pursuing this change vigorously. However, not all have jumped on the bandwagon. I still also find myself uncomfortable with some university leaders' notions of leadership. They make little effort to imbue their management style with empathy and recognition of the other's dignity. Menand sees this as a "tension" and thinks the university is a wonderful place to work out these tensions. We shall see.

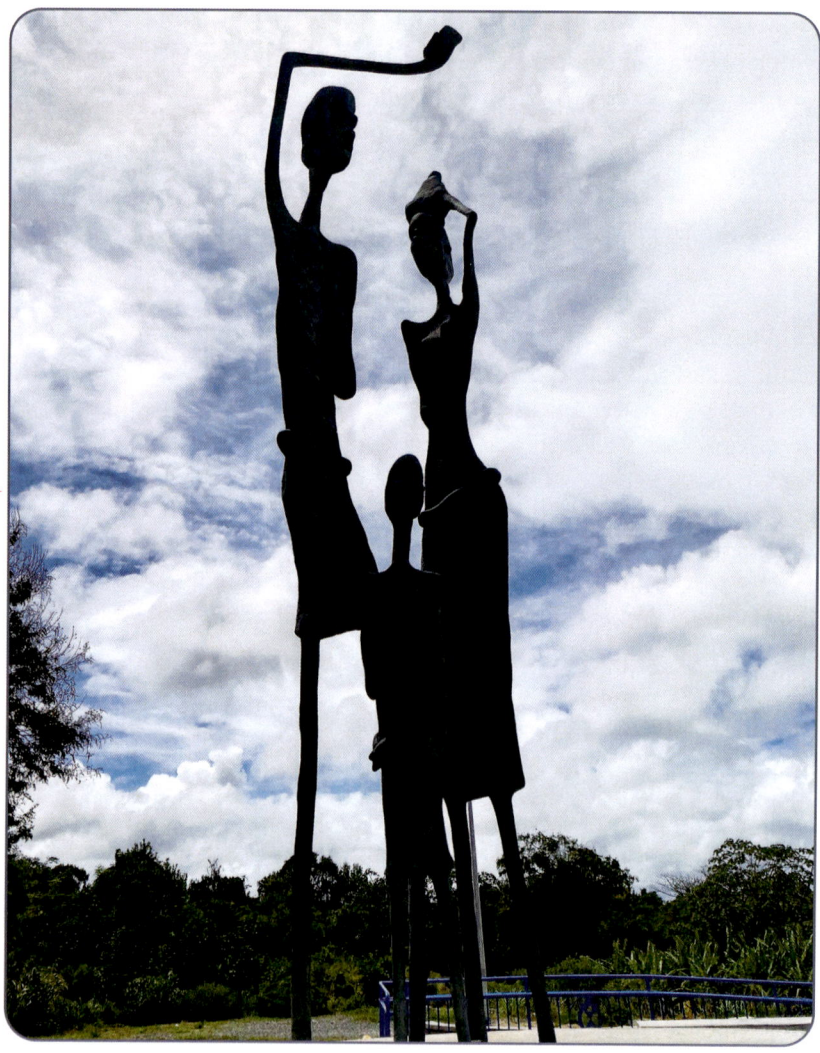

**Figure 1.3** The Rock Hall Monument of Freedom, St. Thomas, Barbados.

Unveiled in August 2005, this public sculpture was designed by Stanton Haynes to represent freedom from mental and physical slavery, guilt, and shame.

*Source.*   Photograph by Brigitte Griffith.

# Comments and Clinical Observations

While growing up in Barbados during the 1950s, I certainly had heard of Black and White people. I was always impressed by how the British were able to create and maintain boundaries that kept Black Barbadians away from Whites without much fanfare or rancor. Elementary school was a sea of Blackness from top to bottom. Occasionally, I encountered a solitary pupil with a high brown skin that made me wonder about the boy's antecedents. But the event was such a rarity that little attention was paid to him. No such encounters took place in my home village.

Church was a different matter. I grew accustomed to White Anglican priests and the famous British organist and choirmaster who had come to the island a long time ago. In other dimensions of social life, there was the White Canadian family physician. I also quickly developed an inherent recognition, an intuitive understanding that the chief justice of the island, the chief of police, the Lord Bishop, and of course the governor (representing England's reigning monarch) were most likely to be White. There was a naturalness to that reality, unquestioned by anyone within my hearing, which made it seem ordained by the heavens. The policemen I encountered were all Black, except for the few senior officers, and so were my Sunday school teachers and scout leaders. Life was balanced and orderly; my young life seemed largely unfettered, straightforward, ordinary, and predictable.

Much later, I would learn that World War II had ended in 1945. And then I would realize that a strange notion of freedom was circulating throughout the Caribbean that would lead to the island's independence from Britain in 1966. In 1950s Barbados, adults were more concerned about having a job and being able to feed their families. We children appeared somewhat protected from the iniquities of poverty and disparities, even as our parents worked hard to absorb, on our behalf, the maleficence of colonialism. Payback time would, of course, come in later years. I did not grow up close to a sugar plantation, and I knew little about that life of brutal manual labor in the hot sun. Everyone in my village was familiar with poverty, but the children felt it without the malignant accompanying features of indignity and persistent persecution.

However, there was the occasional experience that came, with the passage of time, to be an explicit irritant. It occurred from time to time at my favorite beach where I would go with friends and without parental supervision. I imagined that the expanse of sand was certainly among the most beautiful anywhere in the world. Relatively flat and creamy-white, with the water lapping gently at the edge, we youngsters romped and screamed and wrestled with each other. The Europeans were there because that is where their aquatic and yacht clubs were built. The beach belonged to no private entity, which did not stop the clubs' owners from claiming that the beaches abutting their clubs were also private property. They hired what we called "watchmen" to keep us Black youngsters off their beach. That was my first confrontation, my up-close interaction with Black-White difference. The transaction did not imply that I was in danger. There could not even have been, within the interior of the incident, a suggestion that Whites were superior to Black people. That was impossible because I was a good athlete, competed readily and effectively at school, and lived in a house where parents made clear that we children had status. I believe now that the most important lesson had to do with Whites' sense of entitlement and privilege. They asserted the right to take what they wanted and to cover up their behavior with artifice and deceit. And to be truthful, they did it, in Barbados, in my time, without violence.

In 1956, my family would make the unsurprising move to New York's Brooklyn. My colleagues like to call this an act of displacement, which it was. My entire family felt the uprootedness and risk implicated in these moves. Still, we knew that migration was a common occurrence among West Indian families. Employment and economic opportunities were relatively rare in the small Caribbean islands. Thus, a geographic move was always a possibility. An important dimension to the move was that it highlighted what our parents had constructed in the Barbadian home-space: the tight-knit safety and security of the space, the distinctive smells of Caribbean cuisine, the laughter and children's games everywhere, the coming and going of neighbors borrowing or sharing something, and the stories being heard or told as my mother leaned out a window in conversation with neighbors all fell apart with the move. What we had in Barbados was a nest, a place in which ideas of home and belonging percolated.

None of us knew, while living in Barbados, what the characteristics of a satisfying home-space were. Once we arrived in New York, however, we understood what we had lost. I recognize now that an important protective feature of my Barbadian household was the combined leadership and supervision of my parents. My mother ran a house that placed her six children's welfare up front. In our village, everyone knew her, and she enjoyed a peculiar form of deep respect. She had no role to play in being militant about anything. She had no desire to overturn any of the mundane practices that defined the routine of our home.

In Barbados, one day, a policeman knocked on our door inquiring whether he could talk to me about a fight that had taken place the night before at a church. My mother stood up to him with a confidence that surprised even the constable. Nobody could question one of her children just like that. First, I had a father, and she had a husband. And then, there were lawyers. There are other stories I could recount about my father and his responses to people, both White and Black. He would take us to a Saturday afternoon football match and people would greet him left and right. That included all ranks and classes of individuals. He was always respectful, while staying fearless. With little money in his pocket, he acted as though he was close friends of those who controlled the sports venue.

Elsewhere (Griffith 2018, p. 150), I described, in relation to geographic moves from one place to another, the inordinate suffering that can accompany displacement and mobility. I talked, too, of Michael Rowe's notion of the sort of metamorphosis that can occur in the context of migration (Rowe 2002). Movement north to New York rendered everything precarious, and it transformed identity into a tool that was frail and always dependent on the support of others. That external aid was mercifully there, from friends, church, relatives, and other unlikely sources. I believe all of us also became attuned to this new idea of a peculiar caste system in the United States built on racial discrimination. Everyone talked about it in Brooklyn, all through the next several decades, and from all angles. I was too young to appreciate race matters fully. But adults around me kept up their tutorial sessions.

I attended a high school that, although ensconced amidst a Black community, had a long record of producing talented graduates. The school had three different streams of curriculum. For some reason, a teacher came to me one day and said that he would recommend that I be moved into the scholarship group. There, I found some excitement. I enjoyed the frequent essays and the reading list. Many of the books I have long forgotten. But not Richard Wright's *Native Son*. From that, I stumbled upon other literary members of the Harlem Renaissance, and a world of unexplored books opened to me. I gradually became sensitive to this matter of difference, racial difference. Of course I had long been aware of skin-color contrasts. But that was more along the lines of aesthetic preferences. It never crossed my mind that anyone would seriously argue that certain groups from birth could be considered inherently inferior to other groups. Even in Brooklyn at that time, my family physician was a Black Barbadian who had trained at the University of Edinburgh. However, the violence in *Native Son* put everything in a different light. References to the Black/White dichotomy seemed more common and a topic of serious and passionate conversations.

As I looked around me, it was clear that I quickly established affective connections to Barbadian immigrants who were in my school. We went together to the same parties on weekends and church services on Sunday evenings. We were teammates on the school soccer team. People of other nationalities were on the team as well, but they went off on their own once practice was over. I noticed cultural differences emerging. In class, some White students talked excitedly of Broadway and the latest productions going on there. My group chatted about the recent orchestra appearing at the Palladium, the Manhattan home of Latin dance music. My buddies and I also flocked after school to the homeroom of a biology teacher who had Caribbean parents. The school ambience felt good, comfortable. The daily rhythms were predictable and enjoyable.

Even as my racialized sensitivity grew, I still would not have understood in the 1950s what Isabel Wilkerson (2020) meant by the notion of a caste system built on oppressive racial discrimination. As a young schoolboy, I had $2 a week for bus fare and lunch money. I had to supplement that from time to time through visits to some adult relative who usually would give me a couple of dollars for pocket money. However, I never had to endure the ignominy of being called names when I entered a store somewhere. Perhaps I missed some of those experiences simply because I had no money to spend on extras. There was simply no reason to enter a store, because actually purchasing an article was not possible. In fact, my father taught me how to go to any sort of gathering with one hand in my pocket and a slight smile on my face that conveyed confidence. He said that once my clothes were clean and pressed, my head held high, and my vocal responses unhurried and grammatically sound, people would assume that I came from a monied background. He was right. Often, I carried only bus fare.

This idyllic life ceased once I left New York City and went to Harvard to study. This was the early 1960s, and the dining hall conversations were peppered with race talk. There was a steady accumulation of certain facts. Only a small number of Black undergraduates were in my class of about 1,200 students. Nobody talked of African American studies. Still, students knew that off-campus Black fraternities existed, just as there was quiet discussion of the private clubs to which certain Harvard men would seek entrance. That never bothered me at the time because I felt that was just a pale imitation of the business of the aquatic club in Barbados. Nevertheless, a drumbeat with a steady cadence was coming from the discourse of Malcolm X and his exchanges with Martin Luther King Jr. There was tension in the air, and I could feel that White students on campus were becoming concerned about the gradual numerical increase in minorities in the student body as each year went by.

Despite my relatively protected Barbadian upbringing, my exposure to matters of race and caste in Europe and North America over the next several decades certainly provided me a specialized education. The 2 years I spent in the U.S. Army between 1964 and 1966 also provided an extensive tutorial, conducted by young Black men from southern states. They outlined their life experiences and provided their notions of what was possible in their world that was at every turn influenced by their skin color and guided by the engraved principle of their inferiority. It was down-to-earth business, no-holds-barred explication of who "Charlie" (the White man) really was to these folk who had grown up below the Mason-Dixon line. The final 11 months of my military life were an assignment to the Pasteur Institute in Saigon, Vietnam. I had no choice but to reflect on the peculiar irony of my circumstance. I was a participant in research efforts to neutralize the negative effects of plague on the public's health. At the same time, I was part of a military project that pursued a mission of violently imposing its political ideas on a foreign nation.

Between 1967 and 1973, I studied medicine in France, where I soaked up as much as I could about French culture. There, I grasped what that war with Hitler meant to ordinary French citizens. My extended contact with the French also permitted a clearer view of colonial France and the struggles with Algeria. I came to appreciate the French view of its differentiated relationship with the Maghreb as opposed to its interactions with sub-Saharan Africa. I also developed a more informed view of why many Black American artists, after the end of World War II, found solace and shelter in Paris. I was progressively making more sense of my ideas of difference between European and American colonization. The return to the United States and engagement in the academic life provided numerous opportunities to debate matters of race, injustice, and their effect on one's function and self-satisfaction. At the same time, I was sharpening my medical and psychiatric skills and naturally making use of the knowledge and insights acquired in my clinical practice. It is in this context that I approached the columns in this chapter.

In the last 20 years or so, racialized thinking and discourse have had an increasingly powerful effect on the specialized areas of psychiatry and other mental health disciplines. It is now an unavoidable reality; commentators and observers are interested in race matters because race as a sociocultural concept continues to affect multiple arenas of our social world. I say this to advise clinicians that substantial inquiry has been focused on our clinical work. People want to know about the relationship between clinical psychiatry and Black identity; the relevance of the caste notion to what we do; and, for example, whether race plays a role in determining the outcomes of certain treatments. I suggest that a major result of recent scholarly inquiry in our profession is recognition that what goes on in the social world may affect our mental health and general well-being. In the last few years, I have spent considerable time with White clinicians discussing race matters. A recurring dilemma for them has been a fear of posing questions about race to patients belonging to non-White groups. Another difficulty that came to light was staying clinically neutral in discussions about the Gaza and Ukraine conflicts. Expressing more empathy toward one group of war victims than another can lead to obvious problems in cross-cultural clinical work.

Take, for example, the first column ("When Diversity Is Not Enough") in this chapter where I discuss diversity and its role in organizational life. I complained that while the term *diversity* has become synonymous with concern about the lack of opportunities for certain groups, attending solely to the problem of diversifying cultural representation will not solve all our problems. I reached that conclusion because my general life experience has taught me that diversity may not mean inclusion. Véronique Griffith (2020) was mindful that we clinicians inherently rely on our familiarity with the concept of biopower to run our medical clinics as we like and extrude certain classes of patients. It is well known that we prefer to treat our good patients. In the column ("Diversity and Curiosity About the Other") where I mentioned Anton Hart's notion of diversity and curiosity, I highlighted his demand that while promoting diversity as a useful tool, we also appreciate the point of experiencing curiosity as we listen with openness. Then, we should concentrate on cultivating an inherent respect for the other. Hart has been pressing for this attitude change in clinicians. I want to tout it also for use by administrators in organizations and different types of organic systems.

This idea of openness toward others is of import and is linked to the task of cultivating a respectful and genuine relationship with our patients. In the context where some form of cultural difference exists between the clinician and the patient, monitoring the connection requires ongoing attention. The lack of a fundamentally trusting interpersonal connection among groups within the APA has highlighted, since at least 1969, the organization's need to improve its internal racialized climate. Christakis (2019) cited this factor's relevance in the functioning of organizations and recommended affection for partners and affinity for one's own group that is not linked to rejection of others. In another column ("Black Identity Politics and Psychiatry"), I noted Shelby's (2007) point that within organizations, we should avoid rhetoric that emphasizes rigidity and power positions as we pursue building community within the multiethnic structure.

I suggest that readers with a clinician's eye should review carefully, as a collective, several columns: the one focused on the Chauvin verdict, White's (2002) theorizing about experiencing hating and actively hating the other, "Talking About Freedom With Louis Menand," and the commentary on Wilkerson's (2020) book *Caste*. Professor Menand uses the historical approach to discuss the notion of freedom, with World War II as a perpetual background. It is an important philosophical exercise as well. However, Wilkerson uses a microscope to examine freedom at a granular level, to see how expectations of inferiority are set in place in a way that affects how people are treated and forced to live. When applied to the United States, the caste system also establishes the notion of White privilege. Kathleen White (2002) makes clear that the mixture of caste and privilege is toxic and can produce the Chauvin phenomenon through the mechanism of White police brutality. Other clinical theorists have been discussing the potential for the Black victims, too, to react violently. White suggests that clinicians must learn to talk about hate in the clinical context, to air it out, and to contemplate their own possible contribution to the phenomenon.

## Questions to Ponder

1. Are Black clinicians entitled to a set of ethics principles that differ from those of White clinicians?
2. Black people seeking change and equality in a predominantly White organization may find themselves caught between taking rigid power positions and promoting community. What would you recommend they do?
3. Some scholars have taken the position that White privilege and superiority should be called a European-American psychosis. What do you think of that idea?
4. Should curiosity and openness replace diversity as a reference principle in clinical work?
5. Do Blacks' claims of a unique heritage of suffering justify their demand for Black political solidarity?

## References

Alemu M: Does Chauvin verdict signal real change or is it a mirage? Detroit Free Press, April 21, 2021

Baldwin J: The Fire Next Time. New York, Dial Press, 1963

Blow CM: With the Chauvin verdict, one battle is won: the war continues. New York Times, April 21, 2021

Christakis NA: The Evolutionary Origins of a Good Society. New York, Little, Brown Spark, 2019

Erikson EH: Gandhi's Truth: On the Origins of Militant Nonviolence. New York, WW Norton, 1970

Foucault M: Naissance de la Clinique. Paris, Presses Universitaires, 1963

Griffith EEH: An open letter to black medical students: on belonging at Yale. Yale Psychiatric Quarterly 13:13–15, 1990

Griffith EEH: Belonging, Therapeutic Landscapes, and Networks: Implications for Mental Health Practice. New York, Routledge, 2018

Griffith EEH: The steel pan and decolonizing mental health. Psychiatric News, September 24, 2020

Griffith VAS: Healers and Patients Talk: Narratives of a Chronic Gynecological Disease. Lanham, MD, Lexington Books, 2020

Hart A: Principles of teaching issues of diversity in a psychoanalytic context. Contemp Psychoanal 56(2–3):404–417, 2020

Hickling FW: The European-American psychosis: a psychohistoriographic perspective of contemporary Western civilization. J Psychohist 37(1):67–81, 2009

Menand L: The Free World: Art and Thought in the Cold War. New York, Farrar, Straus & Giroux, 2021

Oshinsky D: Louis Menand examines the churn of American culture after World War II. New York Times Book Review, April 21, 2021

Patterson O: Being and blackness. New York Times Book Review, January 8, 2006

Pazzanese C: Ensuring the Floyd trial becomes a turning point. Harvard Gazette, April 21, 2021

Prograis LJ Jr, Pellegrino ED (eds): African American Bioethics: Culture, Race, and Identity. Washington, DC, Georgetown University Press, 2007

Rowe M: The Book of Jesse: A Story of Youth, Illness, and Medicine. Washington, DC, Francis Press, 2002

Salovey P: Today's verdict on the murder of George Floyd. April 20, 2021. Available at: https://salovey.yale.edu/writings-and-speeches/statements/todays-verdict-murder-george-floyd. Accessed May 27, 2024.

Shelby T: We Who Are Dark: The Philosophical Foundations of Black Solidarity. Cambridge, MA, Harvard University Press, 2007

White KP: Surviving hating and being hated: some personal thoughts about racism from a psychoanalytic perspective. Contemp Psychoanal 38(3):401–422, 2002

Wilkerson I: Caste: The Origins of Our Discontents. New York, Random House, 2020

# 2

# Pursuing Dignity

# Columns From *Psychiatric News*

## Empathy, Compassion, and Dignity in Forensic Psychiatry[1]

Forensic psychiatrists have long been discussing the complex task of carrying out a forensic evaluation and testifying about the results. I contributed to a conversation about this subject in a workshop at the October 2019 annual meeting of the American Academy of Psychiatry and the Law. The moderator, Dr. Sarah Baker of the University of Texas Southwestern Medical School, and two discussants (Dr. Philip Candilis of the George Washington University School of Medicine and Dr. Michael Norko of the Yale School of Medicine) focused on integrating empathy and compassion into forensic evaluation and testimony.

At the outset, Baker framed several questions for our consideration: May an evaluator be said to employ too much empathy or compassion in forensic psychiatry evaluations? Does empathy or compassion add value to the examination? Do those elements pollute the evaluation and compromise forensic psychiatrists' pursuit of objectivity and truth seeking in their work? Besides the problem of potential interference with objectivity, some practitioners worry that empathy and compassion may mislead evaluees into thinking that the evaluator is there as an advocate for those being examined.

Conventional definitions of *empathy* and *compassion* were discussed. For empathy, the "spontaneous feeling of identity with someone who suffers" and "walking in someone's shoes" sufficed. For compassion, there were "kindness," "respect for persons," and "altruism" as helpful explanatory terminology. Two statements emerged clearly from the presentations. Regardless of the approach of forensic psychiatrists to the tasks of evaluation and testimony, evaluees must be allowed to present their concerns and versions of events. In addition, forensic psychiatrists must reflect patiently on managing the integration of empathy and compassion into the work and remain sensitive to potential problems caused by overidentification with evaluees.

In my presentation, I focused on *dignity* as an alternative term to empathy and compassion. Scholars see "dignity" as two-pronged. On

---

[1] Adapted with permission from Griffith EEH: Empathy, Compassion, and Dignity in Forensic Psychiatry. *Psychiatric News*, February 2020. Copyright © 2020 American Psychiatric Association. All rights reserved.

the one hand, it refers to the concept of an internal essential and inviolable humanity, often called *humanitas* or intrinsic dignity. Then there is the dignity imputed to us, referring to our wisdom, rank, and position. This is commonly called *dignitas* or attributed dignity. The ultimate point here was that dignity should be employed thoughtfully in the work of forensic psychiatrists as we strive to interact with evaluees in a dignified fashion.

During the evaluation, for example, how and when does the forensic specialist bring into play considerations of dignity? An artistic exposition recently provided me some insight into this problem. The exhibition took place at the Yale Center for British Art and featured painter Lynette Yiadom-Boakye, who was born in London to Ghanaian parents. Program notes discussed Yiadom-Boakye's objective of making portraits of people of color without their "being considered symbols of pain, suffering, or triumph." In forensic psychiatry, we represent those symbols as we explore the stories of those we evaluate. In addition, this artist talks of stripping "her work of complicated narratives in favor of what the body expresses in stillness, or in action." Consequently, Yiadom-Boakye's paintings present individuals who are "alive with presence and thought." The observer can then see how the models, real or imagined, "display assurance of minds and bodies that are self-contained and exist on their own terms."

This, to my mind, is an effort to recognize intrinsic dignity in the artist's model. Still, it is important to note that building complex narratives about our evaluees is central to our evaluations and should not be forgotten. Can we structure our narratives about our subjects on a foundational core of *humanitas*?

The artist's portraits emphasize the human dimension of people in a visual field of stillness or limited action. I believe this idea comes into play, too, at the beginning of the contact between evaluator and evaluee in forensic work, free for the moment of all ideological concerns. The model reflects the essential and inviolable essence we seek to recognize. We must be calm and patient in seeking the quiet dignity before moving to characterize and bear witness to the complex narrative of the evaluee.

# Memorializing Dignity and Identity in Public Monuments[2]

In late November 2020, just before the Thanksgiving holiday, a friend wrote from Barbados to deliver the long-awaited news. After decades of debate, the island's government had removed the outdoor statue of Vice Adm. Lord Horatio Nelson (1758–1805) to a nearby museum. For over 200 years, it had occupied a central place in the island's Trafalgar Square, opposite the Parliament buildings. Nelson has been hailed as a highly decorated British naval commander, a model of military heroism and tenacity. In recent years, there have been discussions about whether he helped maintain slavery in the British Caribbean islands. Other commentators argued that as a naval officer, it was simply his duty to protect the political economy of Britain, a colonial and slave-holding power at the time.

I still remember from the 1950s a policeman standing on a small circular platform next to the statue directing traffic. He did so with a military precision that made all of us youngsters dream of being so publicly ambidextrous and performative. I recall the arms that moved decisively to control the movement of cars and pedestrians. This was in an area that most of the islanders would pass at least once a week. Nelson was a striking symbol: inscrutable, daring visitors to guess at why he surveyed all before him with such majesty and confidence. Technological advances eventually brought stoplights to the spot, causing the policeman to be superfluous. Nelson stayed on, defying hurricanes and all else, even the island's 1966 independence.

A colleague noted that there is now a recognized defining connection among history, its iconography, and identity. People pose questions pugnaciously about statues, recognizing that they are interrogating themselves and their dignity. Professor Richard Drayton (2016) from King's College London delivered the Sir Winston Scott Memorial Lecture that marked the 50th anniversary of Barbados's independence. In this memorial lecture, Drayton challenged the island's citizens to think about what they were doing with their sovereignty and independence. Drayton acknowledged the island's long history of colonization by Britain that had instilled crippling self-doubt in Barbadians after protracted colonial dependency. He also referred to the international

---

[2] Adapted with permission from Griffith EEH: Memorializing Dignity and Identity in Public Monuments. *Psychiatric News*, January 2021. Copyright © 2021 American Psychiatric Association. All rights reserved.

architecture of White supremacy that Europeans had so studiously put together. In the years following independence, Barbadians took note of developments in the arenas of civil rights, human rights, and protest politics. Eventually, their eyes focused on this statue of Lord Nelson placed so provocatively in their midst next door to their Parliament.

Their questions had to come. They did come. After all, Barbadians read and travel and take stock of what is happening overseas. Museums and different forms of media comment on statues and paintings located in the public sphere. These institutions have been educating us about how these artistic renderings regularly embody special values held dear by their national leadership. We know now that the artistic devices often signify that White supremacy supersedes Black lives in significance. The statue regularly bears witness, borrowing Drayton's expression, to a regimen of economic, social, political, cultural, and spiritual dispossession.

This removing of statues is, of course, not a uniquely Barbadian or Caribbean phenomenon. American universities and governmental agencies have struggled with it for years. The debates have left in their wake some important questions: What moral lessons do the statues convey to the public? Whose heroism do they represent? Who is threatened by them and why? Finally, in the case of Nelson's statue, how did Black parents ever explain its presence to their children?

Today's Barbadians claim that it is time to celebrate native heroes; to build a record of Barbadian achievement; and to dignify the humanity in Barbadians, not the inhumanity of colonial oppression and slavery (see Figure 2.1). As the Caribbean poet Derek Walcott (2004) put it in *The Prodigal*, it is time to memorialize the unimportant beauty of the Caribbean village; to rid ourselves of the envy of European statues; and for Barbadians to feel the humming that so characterizes the tired heart of the West Indian who recognizes that the Caribbean island is truly home.

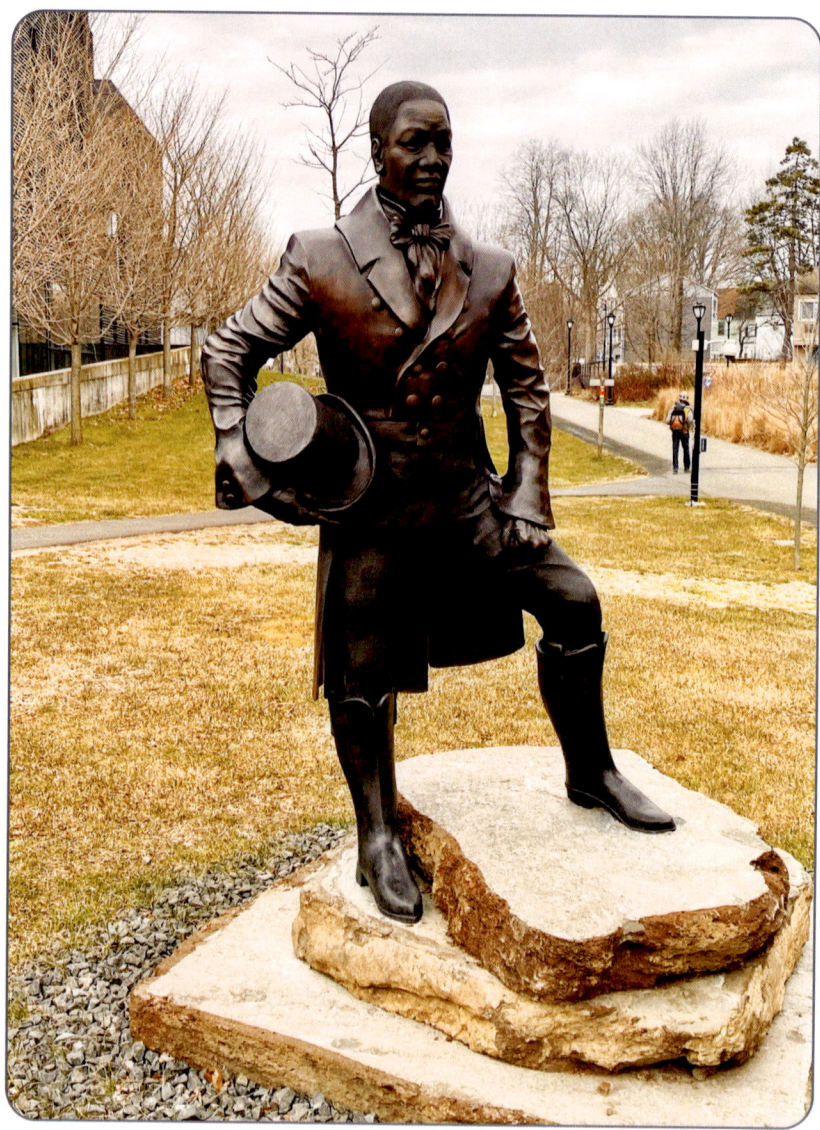

**Figure 2.1** Statue of William Lanson by Dana King, New Haven, Connecticut.

It was dedicated on September 26, 2020. Lanson (~1782–1851) was a master builder who constructed the Liberian Hotel in the middle of New Haven, Connecticut. A Black freeman known for his participation in community projects, his clothing and bearing give him a dignified air.

*Source.*   Photograph by Brigitte Griffith.

# Identity and Political Independence[3]

On November 30, 2021, my 166 square miles of island, known to the initiated as Bimshire and to others as Barbados, became a republic. I read about it in English, French, and American newspapers and imagined it had even wider coverage. Friends wrote to congratulate me, claiming it was a notable event. Others described the accompanying celebrations, expected me to be pleased by the news, and asked how things would be different now. Professor Richard Drayton (2021), a historian at King's College London and an expert in the long relationship between Barbados and the United Kingdom, commented on the Caribbean island's journey to becoming a republic.

Drayton explained that following Barbados's independence from Britain in 1966, the winds of what he called "the Black Power moment" buffeted the Caribbean islands in the 1970s. The result was that Guyana, Trinidad and Tobago, and Dominica took the status of a republic. For several reasons, Barbados did not follow this trend and remained in the British Commonwealth with Queen Elizabeth as head of state. However, the island's political leaders did make changes after independence that suggested they were keeping an eye on becoming a republic. Professor Drayton buttressed this point with examples: The island's Anglican Church was disestablished and disendowed in 1969, putting that faith group on its own fiscal bottom and disentangling the connections between church and state. In 1972, the Central Bank of Barbados took over fiscal policy. At the turn into the 21st century, Barbados replaced its reliance on the Judicial Committee of the Privy Council and agreed that the new Caribbean Court of Justice should be its highest appellate court. The Caribbean Court of Justice was inaugurated in 2005. Drayton's examples indicated a steady maturing of Barbados's intention to fracture the ties to the mother country. Nevertheless, some palpable hesitancy remains among some of the island's citizens about this new status that dispenses with the queen as their head of state.

Judging from his other writing, Drayton (2016) understood that the 1966 independence was only a first step toward economic, cultural, spiritual, and psychological decolonization. In a certain sense, this new phase of becoming a republic should be viewed as a marker of entrance into what Drayton sees as secondary decolonization. We Barbadians,

---

[3] Adapted with permission from Griffith EEH: Identity and Political Independence. *Psychiatric News*, February 2022. Copyright © 2022 American Psychiatric Association. All rights reserved.

at home and in the diaspora, must cease being self-alienated. It should be obvious that building a postcolonial future that is closely linked to British interests is not true independence. Drayton (2021) acknowledged that most Barbadians did support the move to become a republic; however, it was not a position passionately held. He worried that some citizens may not even have understood what was in the decision and what it meant for the lives of those "on the underside of the society, living on biscuits, rice, and a little corned beef." He was not confident that there was broad understanding of "what the Republic is for" or in what ways it is truly ours.

My own observations confirm Drayton's, and I turn to a cynical preoccupation of mine. Some Barbadians, likely among elders, remain enamored of British royalty and hopeful that for the foreseeable future they will be protected by a lingering magical connection to their beloved queen. Jamaican Professor Frederick Hickling (2021) tried mightily to help West Indians confront their history of slavery and oppression at the hands of the British. He thought that the British exploitation of Caribbean Blacks stemmed from a psychological belief that European colonizers were inherently superior to the colonized. Hickling's work is clearly now an antecedent to the present reflections of American psychoanalysts on the theme of White privilege and superiority. For example, Donald Moss (2021) was concerned about how this sense of superiority could become an instrument of power. The more one exercised dominion power, the more one became certain and confident in its implementation. Moss applied his theorizing to understanding better how and why the developed countries of the world treated so shamefully those who were still in the process of developing. Of course, we know that similar ideas have been articulated about France's colonial involvement in Algeria and other countries. Hickling wanted Caribbean peoples to give up mimicking the White colonizers and to develop pride and confidence in Caribbean traditions. This is plainly a part of Drayton's idea of secondary decolonization.

Hickling and Moss understood the impact of images imposed by enslavers and colonizers on their victims' psyches. Barbados has made significant strides between 1966 and 2021. Still, its citizens must think carefully about their new political status and their own worth. It is not an easy task, as I am talking about an improvement in personal and group identity. However, the island is well supplied, at home and throughout the diaspora, with insightful individuals who can point the way to a deeper sense of confidence and self-reliance. We are people, too.

# The Justice and Affirmative Action[4]

For a long time, I have thought that writing about single lives is at the heart of what my friend and colleague Yale Professor Michael Norko (2018) calls "vocation." In this case, the term would refer to the spirituality that resides within the composing of biographies. Norko has explored different definitions of what one might mean by spirituality in a specific context. One that I like concerns doing what is in the interest of others and oneself. Norko was aware that God is not mentioned in that definition, yet he concluded that we must consider the meaning of spirituality that is related to our daily work, which then brings us to the subject of vocation.

This brief exposition of Norko's *vocation* has guided my examination of biographical writing. I always want to understand how the subject approached life; the expressed relatedness to others; the salience of work, of play; the practical application of effort and time to specific activities; the connection between love of neighbor and service through one's profession; the image of self as represented in one's work and personal actions.

It is with Michael Norko in mind that I settled down to reading the *New York Times Magazine* article by Danny Hackim and Jo Becker (2018): "The Long Crusade of Clarence and Ginni Thomas." It is a detailed, complex piece about a current Supreme Court justice and his wife. Both are ardent conservatives who enjoy the limelight as leaders of the anti-libertarian movement in this country. I concentrate here only on Clarence Thomas's view that affirmative action undercuts self-reliance. I have no interest at all in his personal health, and I have never met him.

We learn from Thomas's biographers that he was raised by his grandfather in the South and graduated from the College of the Holy Cross. From there, he attended Yale Law School. It appears that graduation did not bring prestigious job offers. In addition, some individuals apparently suggested that his acceptance to Yale was based on preferential treatment. In other words, he may have been a token Yale student, pulled from the line of Black applicants and pushed ahead because of his minority status. Those Yale years became an important event in Thomas's life. From then, he matured into a zealous anti–affirmative

---

[4] Adapted with permission from Griffith EEH: The Justice and Affirmative Action. *Psychiatric News*, April 2022. Copyright © 2022 American Psychiatric Association. All rights reserved.

action ambassador, with a will to destroy the affirmative action movement. Of course, there are others intent on accomplishing that objective. However, Thomas's voice carries weight. People listen to him when he speaks. He also knows, because many have praised him in public, that he has access to distinguished social groups that grant few Blacks entrance, and his presence is distinctive.

I understand that suggesting he benefited from affirmative action may have left him disappointed, less authoritative than he wanted to be. Only he knows, of course. But why would he dismantle a mechanism that has served so many others in past years? His biographers did not mention whether he has a replacement for affirmative action. I am curious about this point. I wonder how he thinks about these things. Education is linked to mental health. When access to educational institutions is circumscribed and identity development is limited, so is generous access to excellence.

I anticipate the suggestion that it is not the jurist's role to find solutions to sociopolitical dilemmas. However, as we all know, that is an antiquated principle. Many professions have tried out that excuse, including the medical profession, to no useful end. Jurists these days must be aware of their decisions' effects on neighbors. I return to Norko's comments on the link between spirituality and vocation. I just wish I could see the interest in others, the love of neighbor that the Justice brings to these debates. Affirmative action does not undercut self-reliance. Such a claim mocks efforts at self-improvement.

## Expanding the Limits of Empathy[5]

Professor Peter Brooks (2006), the interdisciplinary Yale scholar with an acute interest in narrative, has cautioned us about the problem of perspective in stories. He appreciated fully storytelling's role in our quest to understand human beings and their behaviors. He also grasped the potential of narrative to mislead. Brooks' cautions come alive whenever I read press reports of important events, such as the tragic school shooting in Uvalde, Texas. We wake up commonly enough these days to all forms of media announcing what has happened: the violence, the gratuitous loss of life, the waste of human and material resources, and

---

[5] Adapted with permission from Griffith EEH: Expanding the Limits of Empathy. *Psychiatric News*, August 2022. Copyright © 2022 American Psychiatric Association. All rights reserved.

the ritualized putting-on of sackcloth and ashes to atone for our failure to find solutions. In the face of these crises, narratives take on urgency. Many of the narrators claim objectivity and neutrality. When those who have suffered are children, it is understandable that the nation comes together and worries. Eventually, political interests formulate polarizing suggestions that primarily protect their territory, while striving to dominate the discourse and leave untouched the heart of the violence problem.

In reviewing the Texas school incident, I did not work very hard at recognizing the plethora of positions concerning access to weapons and maintenance of schools as safe spaces devoid of guns. I had considerable practice at this when I served on the commission examining the Sandy Hook School shooting in Connecticut. This is what characterizes the marketplace following these tragic events. There are many people from all walks of life commenting on a variety of elements from a multitude of vantage points. They follow the traditions of narrators, coloring the stories to reach certain objectives. I make no condemnations of this practice; I simply draw attention to the obvious: It is common in the reporting of events. After all, Brooks has told us that narrative is perspectival. Despite this bustle of activity and the significant effort expended to describe the context of each school event, there often seems to be modest inquiry about the perpetrator. In fact, I have noted efforts to obliterate their identities, with accompanying claims that making these perpetrators visible in any way is a misguided celebration of their deeds.

There is another technique for dealing with the perpetrators, described by Gwen Adshead, a forensic psychiatrist and colleague. She has talked about our penchant for creating "monster stories," a term that I simply cannot stop from coming into view as I read accounts of these school shootings. In other words, do these individuals have any redeeming features? Is there any aspect of humanity in them? Do they resemble us in any way? In my experience with the aftermaths of these events, I have recognized that, for several reasons, the stories about the perpetrators are generally incomplete and, in Brooks' terms, not sufficiently plausible. There are specialized ethics rules and general societal dictates that account for some of this. I wonder whether there are other impediments to engaging with some modest theorizing about them. I think we are afraid of seeing any of ourselves in them or even recognizing that social and biological elements play some part, even if modest, in the creation of these individuals.

Adshead is the author of a book with Eileen Horne (2021) about people who commit horrific acts of violence, whom we can easily classify as monsters. In its introduction, Adshead offers the invitation to read about these people, to give up our fear, denial, or intolerance of them. She concedes readily that it will demand of us a sort of radical empathy. She acknowledges that we may well ask whether the subjects have any right to feeling love, sorrow, or even regret. She assures the reader, nevertheless, that taking the dive will lead to understanding people as individuals, not as points of information or mythological elements.

The excursion may well transform our lives. Adshead suggests that getting a closer look at those who cause such havoc in our communities may cause an expansion of the limits of empathy. We may then recognize humanity in them and sprinkle greater compassion in our reactions to the baffling events they produce. My hope is that increasing authenticity and authorial responsibility in these narratives about community violence might lead to solutions that benefit the community.

## Making Choices on a Journey[6]

On the last Sunday in July 2022, I attended the 10:00 A.M. service at the Friendship Baptist Church in Atlanta, Georgia. I was in the company of a longtime psychiatrist friend, Professor Quentin Ted Smith. It was a joyous reunion in the precincts of his home church. I had no idea that Morehouse and Spelman colleges took form in the basement of Friendship Baptist sometime in the 1860s. However, the faith group presently occupies an imposing multifunction modern structure dedicated in July 2017. Dr. Smith and I had become good friends over the years, and I was curious about his recent activities. I considered him one of the tranquil and effective sages in American psychiatry. He was not garrulous about his talents or his deeply generous spirit. He is vice chair of education in the Department of Psychiatry at the Morehouse School of Medicine (Figure 2.2). I believe that we first met years ago at a conference organized by the Black Psychiatrists of America. I had not seen him since I was the guest speaker at a white coat ceremony about 20 years ago at Morehouse.

---

[6] Adapted with permission from Griffith EEH: Making Choices on a Journey. *Psychiatric News*, October 2022. Copyright © 2022 American Psychiatric Association. All rights reserved.

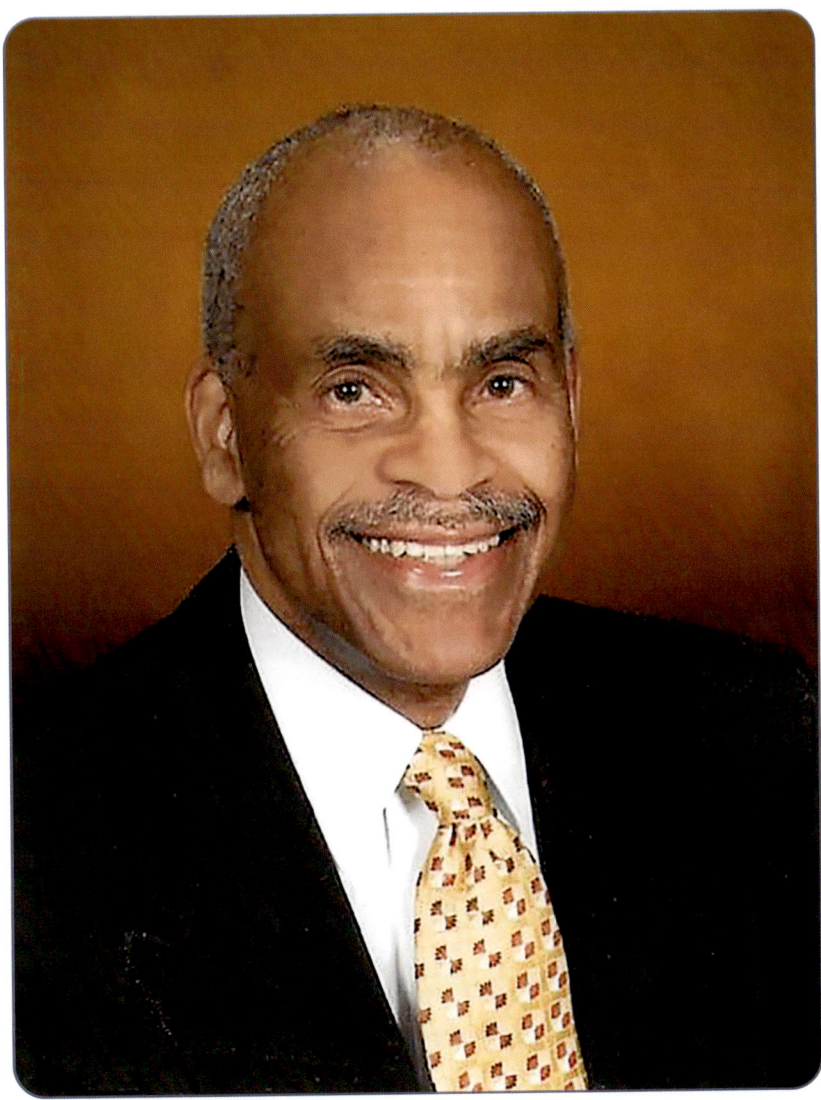

**Figure 2.2** Quentin Ted Smith, M.D.

He is a professor of psychiatry and vice chair of education in the Morehouse School of Medicine, Department of Psychiatry.

*Source.* Photograph provided by Quentin Ted Smith, M.D.

I learned that Dr. Smith was a member of the choir slated to sing that Sunday. He was attired, like the other male singers, in a dark suit with a white silk tie and white shirt. Since he is still a half-marathoner and long-distance walker in his 9th decade, he fit into the suit with an understated elegance. He could gain admission to most church choirs anywhere because, as a college undergraduate, he sang first tenor with the Fisk University Jubilee Singers. That is a distinction few can claim. Later, at lunch, he explained that the Black church had long occupied a central space in his life. His music, he said, speaks to others, as does the calligraphy he employs in the letters he pens to members in his church who are grieving loss.

His parents raised him in Brooklyn, New York, where he grew up in the Kingsboro projects. He attended Franklin K. Lane High School and then enrolled at Hunter College, one of the sections of the City University of New York. He felt a bit disheartened by the experience. He seemed to be missing the magic he wanted from the combination of home and school. The Yale psychologist Miraj Desai (2014) suggests that such feelings sometimes prompt us to renounce being sedentary and to travel outside our usual confines to seek change. By chance, friends who knew about Fisk University encouraged young Ted Smith to make the move, to take a different fork in the road and travel South. These unexpected encounters can produce decision-making that leads to the most special of places.

I did not ask him whether at that point he was familiar with Robert Frost's 1915 poem, "The Road Not Taken." However, his moving to Fisk turned out to make all the difference in his life. Others have also told me stories about how historically Black colleges enter people's lives and turn things around. He clearly appreciated the intellectual curiosity of this concentrated collection of Black people on a single campus. He was carried away by the wave of positivity and the constructive use of time, place, and energy. Everyone seemed focused, intent on achieving something. He could see it just in the way the students walked. And the professors took the time to be helpful and considerate. From his discourse, I could tell that he models some of his pedagogical style on what he witnessed at Fisk. After the first semester, he was awarded a scholarship. His performance earned him a place in Phi Beta Kappa in his senior year.

He graduated in 1961 and spent a year pursuing a Ph.D. at the University of Chicago in biopsychology. He missed the culture, the interactions, the spirit that had emerged so powerfully at Fisk. He took a year off and reoriented himself toward medicine. Robert Frost was right. It serves little purpose to stay on a disappointing pathway and brood. Alternatively, as a single traveler, he could not stay on more than one road at the same time. Frost makes clear, in his famous 1915 poem "The Road Not Taken," that such simultaneity is not permitted: "Two roads diverged in a yellow wood, And sorry I could not travel both…" So, Dr. Smith enrolled at the Howard University College of Medicine and found a new home. In it, he established the habits and rituals that Professor Devika Chawla (2015) says can restore a person into himself.

Professor Smith completed his medical studies in 1967, loving the experience and noting that his teachers were fantastic. By 1973, he completed specialty training in general and in child and adolescent psychiatry. He taught at Emory University School of Medicine before moving to Morehouse in 1984, where both he and his pathologist wife would build careers as celebrated master teachers and scholars. He modeled the physician role for his charges. Unlike many, he stayed away from administration because it often seemed to carry too much of a "misery index." He preferred the interactions with trainees curious about healing and caring for others.

He uses the solitude and isolation of his long walks and leisurely promenades around the city to think and recharge his energy. He has enjoyed remarkable privileges in life and has few regrets about his routine choices. Whenever presented with the dilemma of confronting two roads, he took one, recognizing that a choice is simply mandatory. I came away from our encounter repeating the poet Walt Whitman's lines from "To Think of Time" (Subsection from "Leaves of Grass"): "Something long preparing and formless is arrived and form'd in you, You are henceforth secure, whatever comes or goes."

## The Long Journey From Arigbawonwo[7]

There are many published stories of international medical graduates settling in the United States. A good collective example is described by Daniel José Gastambide (2019) in his *A People's History of Psychoanalysis*. He discusses the early psychoanalysts fleeing persecution in Europe and seeking safety on this side of the pond. The account is grand by design, signaling the historicity of psychoanalysis. However, there are

---

[7] Adapted with permission from Griffith EEH: The Long Journey from Arigbawonwo. *Psychiatric News*, March 2023. Copyright © 2023 American Psychiatric Association. All rights reserved.

quieter tales of this search for refuge, like the one I recount here about the Nigerian Dr. Joel Akande Idowu (Figure 2.3). His story is about being caught in the mundane pressures of life in a developing country that offers minimal opportunities to bloom and flourish. The local conditions often just favor migration, one of the most common outlets for releasing social and economic pressure in one's homeland. A subsequent life focus is to explore the possibility of putting down roots in a foreign land.

Joel Idowu was the youngest of five siblings born to a farmer father and trader mother in Arigbawonwo (pronounced Aree-ba-won-wó), a hamlet of about 200 citizens located in Ogun State in western Nigeria. There were no formal birth certificates issued there, although Joel's father kept a ledger that recorded important birth events. Growing up in that village made Joel noticeable because of his innate curiosity and cheerful disposition that collectively suggested a youngster with academic promise. He also had older cousins who were schoolteachers. They kept an eye on him and obtained his father's permission to take responsibility for Joel's education. The schoolteachers moved around the region from one job to another to improve their professional status. So, they soon realized that maintaining continuity in Joel's education would require his placement in a boarding school. That happened in 1973, and Joel became a boarding student at age 12. When his father died in 1975, an older relative took over defraying the cost of Joel's education.

The boarding school had its advantages, and Joel flourished in the new context. The students, all boys, came from a wider community and from families that were Muslim, Catholic, or Protestant. English was the language of instruction, but Yoruba remained the medium of discourse at home. He was also exposed to Islamic religious instruction and to the Arabic language. He enjoyed being the best student in class and became more outgoing in the comfortable school environment. The long vacations were for spending time with his mother. This divided life was pleasurable and suited his disposition.

Joel's solid academic performance justified his relatives' financial support and reassured him that he was not wasting the generous outlay of money spent on him. When he was ultimately admitted to the University of Lagos in 1982 as a medical student, he saw himself moving among future doctors from families accustomed to privilege. He had no stories to tell about the benefits of being born with the proverbial silver spoon securely placed in his mouth. He realized in medical

*Pursuing Dignity*

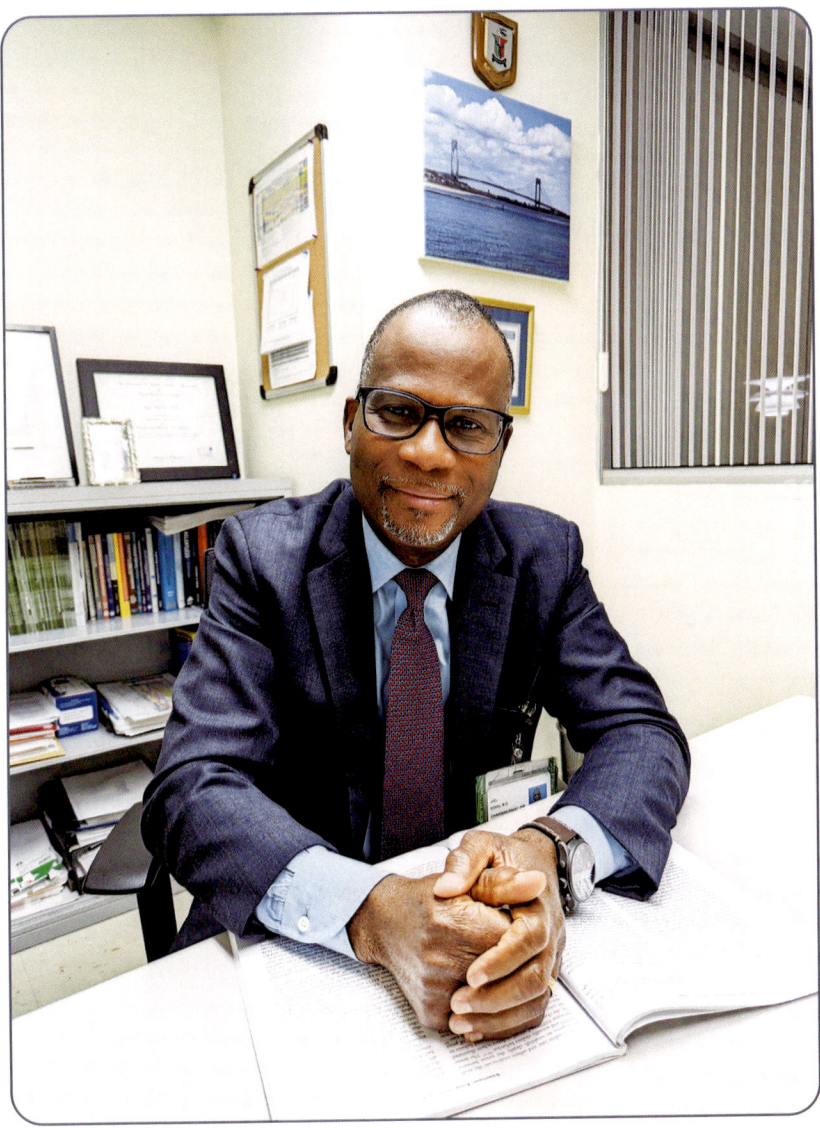

**Figure 2.3**  Joel Idowu, M.D.

A native of western Nigeria, Idowu chairs the Department of Psychiatry at Richmond University Medical Center, Staten Island, New York.

*Source.*   Photograph provided by Joel Idowu, M.D.

school that it would be worthwhile for him to become adept at student politics and to think about matters such as leadership, service, and representation of others who lacked a voice in their surroundings.

Joel graduated from medical school in 1987 and went into the required rotating internship in a rural hospital in northern Nigeria. He saw the year as a worthwhile experience learning how to provide medical care with minimal resources. Although frustrating at times, he could sense his increasing clinical sophistication and confidence. This process also helped him recognize that he had no social or family connections that could help him set up a medical practice in Nigeria. Thus, the most viable option was to migrate overseas and obtain postgraduate training in Europe or North America. He accepted the pathway of a 2-year contract with the Trinidad government. At the end of that, his wife was recruited by a New York City hospital. It was she who obtained the visas that facilitated resettlement in the United States in 1992. It then took him another 2 years to win a place in the psychiatry residency program at Harlem Hospital. After that, he specialized in forensic psychiatry at the State University of New York in Syracuse.

Over the next 15 years, he moved through both inpatient and outpatient hospital positions and finally reached a senior post leading the Department of Psychiatry at New York City's Richmond University Medical Center. His major roles as a clinician educator and physician executive reflect the benefits of his experiences with mundane impediments and barriers to smooth success. I often contemplate his deft manner of handling an administrative meeting or his distinguished performance as an expert witness in court and marvel at the long journey from the Nigerian hamlet to the pinnacle of his present profession. I wonder at the elements that nourish such resilience and accomplishment.

## When Outsiders Come In[8]

On my recent visit to London's Victoria and Albert Museum, there were waves of people moving back and forth, sure of where they were going. Art occupied every inch of space as far as I could see, the way some rich collectors decorate their salons, refusing to be bound by

---

[8] Adapted with permission from Griffith EEH: When Outsiders Come In. *Psychiatric News*, October 2023. Copyright © 2023 American Psychiatric Association. All rights reserved.

limitations of square footage. This meant the guide was obliged to offer me landmarks to show the zigs and zags I had to make. It was hard to separate discrete rooms from corridors. Everyone seemed delighted to be walled off from outside concerns and enveloped in an arena focused on aesthetics. I liked the feeling of being in a sanctuary with my imagination able to run loose unfettered by limits. No one was worried about missing a train or being late for a meeting. When I reached my destination, another member of the staff recommended I also visit a complementary exhibition called "Between Two Worlds." She thought my needs would be met more effectively there, and she was right.

The focus of this collection was on Francis Williams, a Black Jamaican intellectual born in 1690, and Vanley Burke, also a Black Jamaican. He was born on the island in 1951 and moved to Britain as a young adolescent. The curator's summary suggested that the portraits of the two men, created over 280 years apart, represented reflections on identity, racism, and colonial legacies. Both men are said to have pursued quests for personhood. Burke is well known in the United Kingdom as a photographer and artist. In this exposition, his pictures were on show, illustrating why he has been considered the godfather of Black British photography. His pictures were described as capturing Black presence in Britain, which is now a preoccupation of the art scene in the United Kingdom.

I could see manifestations of this interest as I walked through the museum's corridors and encountered the sculptures of Thomas J. Price. He presented figurative sculptures of Black people's heads, everyday people: taking elements of individuals encountered in the streets of London to create fictional characters. The curator described these figures as psychological portraits intended to influence us to think about status and appearance. Price confronted this problem of who is a subject in European art. The concern is linked to notions of status, social value, and power. I continue to argue that these interconnections led to my reflections on inherent and attributed dignity. Earlier this summer, I noted this theme in an exposition by the American artist Faith Ringgold at the Picasso Museum in Paris. Artists like Price and Ringgold are now mindful of Black presence in the visualization of communities they represent artistically. Art can connect people to certain realities and persuade audiences to contemplate matters of worth and social value.

Given his age, Vanley Burke is a member of the Windrush generation, a group of immigrants from the Caribbean who answered the invitation to move to Britain after World War II and help the mother country get back on its feet. Many traveled to Britain between 1948 and the early 1970s, some of them on a ship named the Empire Windrush. Their treatment at the hands of the British government and its immigration policies provoked a scandal, as the offered welcome turned out to be less than honest. This shook to the core some immigrants' hopes of truly belonging to British society. Consequently, documentation of Blacks' contributions to the mother country over the last 75 years has been a major concern and has been responsible for the flowering of British photographic art and other genres of creativity and observation. Since 2018, June 22 has marked Windrush Day in Britain. The Windrush protest movement has created a special lens through which to view Britain's attitude toward its colonies and its treatment of Blacks who decided to build a future in their new home. Burke's photos bring to life Black Caribbean people in the new adopted spaces: working, studying, loving, hanging out, recreating home, worshipping, resisting, playing, getting a haircut, and debating. At the heart of it all is the quest for good health, prosperity, and self-respect.

I could not reach the end of Burke's display without conjuring up my own journey from Barbados to New York in the mid-1950s. Had anyone followed me with a camera then, the pictures would have produced evidence of my adjusting to school, coping with loss of old friends and acquiring of new ones, learning how to use a bus and a subway, deciphering a new Americanized English, and memorizing the new diplomatic rules governing negotiations with other adolescents. I had to learn about Broadway (as in a Broadway play) and figure out why my new classmates could speak so casually to teachers. I did not even grasp why some of my peers wore three-piece suits to school. My first thought was to ask where the wedding was. There were also the obligations left over from the old country, like my having to visit my mother's aunt, a woman whom I had just met. My mother had me fulfill a duty owed to her relative. That is what Caribbean mothers heaped on their children, following tradition. The aunt generously gave me a dollar or so to recompense my suffering. It was a game they all played.

The time did come when the immigrant in me relaxed in the new surroundings. Despite what we all say about the developed countries, it is often easier to get educated there than back home. And the experiences became more sophisticated. I knew it when I was introduced to the poet Langston Hughes, and I learned about the Harlem Renaissance. Talk about widening horizons for outsiders who get in!

# That Music From Overseas[9]

The current political discourse encompasses, for some people, a strident call for exclusion of others who come from overseas. The dicta, explicit and implicit, suggest that we foreign born have nothing or little to offer in just about any sphere of life. The irony and madness in this claim always shock me because of its obvious falsity. I have lived long enough in France to say to its extreme right politicians that if we removed their talented foreign masons, carpenters, and painters from France, the country would collapse. A similar thing would happen if we sent away all the foreign taxi drivers, nurses, police, and physicians currently working in the United States. Instead of settling down to organizing a thoughtful immigration system, why do politicians find it easier to lie about us "others" and claim that many of us are simply subhuman? Why can't we find a structured and workable openness to foreign others? We might have a chance if we started listening to the music from other countries.

I recently attended a musical program focused on Ethiopian classical music. It was my first experience with a public offering of East African music. Luckily for me, I was seated next to an Ethiopian woman who helped me understand the structure of the evening's program at New York City's Carnegie Hall. The concert was performed by Girma Yifrashewa, one of the country's distinguished classical pianists. He gave a title to his performance: "Peace Unto Ethiopia: An Anthology of Original Works and Tributes." He and other dignitaries at the celebration talked of using music to pull people together. There was also a collective emphasis on peace instead of war. They underlined a third idea: It was important for all countries to have their own music.

My Ethiopian neighbor reprised this point during the intermission and expanded on it, articulating the pride that many immigrants exude when discussing essential characteristics of the former home space. In fact, she took pleasure in stating clearly that Ethiopia had never been colonized. When I asked about the history of Italy's presence in the country, she repeated firmly that no one had colonized her country. Italy's presence was an occupation. The implication was that Ethiopia had withstood the occupation, conserved its dignity, and built an East African identity impregnable to European interference. I liked this

---

[9] Adapted with permission from Griffith EEH: That Music From Overseas. *Psychiatric News*, August 2024. Copyright © 2024 American Psychiatric Association. All rights reserved.

woman's insistence on representing herself and native country, arguing at every step in the manner of those who enjoy quietly resisting the pressures of cultural colonization. She recognized that for some reason, she had engaged in displacement, to migrate away from home. She was still holding on to the indigenous.

The concert itself debuted with a piece dedicated to Emaboy Tsegué-Mariam Guèbrou, a nun of the Ethiopian Orthodox Church who pioneered Ethiopian classical music. Readers may be interested in *The New Yorker* article in which Amanda Petrusich (2023) discussed the life and work of this personage. I learned that Guèbrou was born on December 12, 1923, and died at age 99. She is said to have been influenced by the Western classical canon and ancient liturgical chants. Petrusich (2023) described Guèbrou's piano artistry as soothing and meditative, with the capacity to soften, and evoking the delicacy of early spring. I note that those words, applied by Petrusich to Guèbou, came from an experienced music critic. I found that the description fitted well my own reactions to "The Shepherd With the Flute," which Yifrashewa played in honor of the nun.

The other Ethiopian piano compositions performed by the evening's guest artist were melodies reflecting the peacefulness of sleep, celebrating laughter, conveying spiritual messages, and transmitting joy and happiness. It was not at all surprising that a segment of the program included European composers like Chopin, Eric Satie, and Debussy. I knew that Yifrashewa would be tempted to demonstrate his accomplished artistry by tackling the Europeans. I admit, too, I was curious about how he would treat them. I concluded that he was outstanding with the non-Ethiopian composers I knew. I felt like belting out some ululation, which is what my neighbor and many others did throughout the concert. They claimed this pianist as theirs, reveled in a bit of home, and said to the world, "We have good musicians too."

# Comments and Clinical Observations

My interest in the concept of human dignity has grown during the last decade. I am persuaded that dignity and indignity play powerful roles in the daily lives of people and their communities. We all yearn for status, recognition, and the comfort of feeling that we have worth. We are also upset by the repeated experience of indignity. When I refer to human dignity, I have in mind the notion defined by Daniel Sulmasy (2013). Dignity generally means something about the worth, stature, or value of an individual. Edmund Pellegrino (2008) used similar terminology, calling human dignity estimations of one's personal worth and worthiness. The subject has gained substantial currency over the last two decades in the biomedical sphere. Scholars have been shedding light on the concept, while ethicists have been worrying about indignities being perpetrated in a variety of medical contexts, especially in prisons and secure hospital facilities. In politics, dignity has been a consideration for as long as people have been talking seriously about values such as freedom, equality, autonomy, and independence—what Jeannette Pols (2013a, p. 188) has called "citizen values."

Dignity is often encountered in community spaces, linked to public art and sculpture. We see it in politics and public policy, exhibited by leaders of educational institutions, and reflected in the decision-making and organizational life of many companies. Military organizations boast of protecting the dignity of their prisoners, and our courts insist that the dignity of those who seek their help be protected. Dignity is therefore a ubiquitous and fundamental theme in our clinical work. Readers will note here the importance of dignity in the columns collected in this chapter.

It is helpful to outline some other elements related to human dignity. Sulmasy, Pellegrino, and Pols, cited earlier, subscribed to the notion that, for practical purposes, dignity is best understood as separable into two categories. *Intrinsic dignity* refers to the value that we have simply by being human. *Attributed dignity* describes the worth or status that we confer on ourselves or others (see Figure 2.4). Intrinsic dignity, then, is inviolable. It cannot be lessened or eliminated by any means. It entitles us to human rights and freedoms and is regularly mentioned in governmental constitutions and declarations. Therefore, when we attempt to label certain groups as inferior to us, we are really trying to attribute a certain worth, value, or merit to the group, which

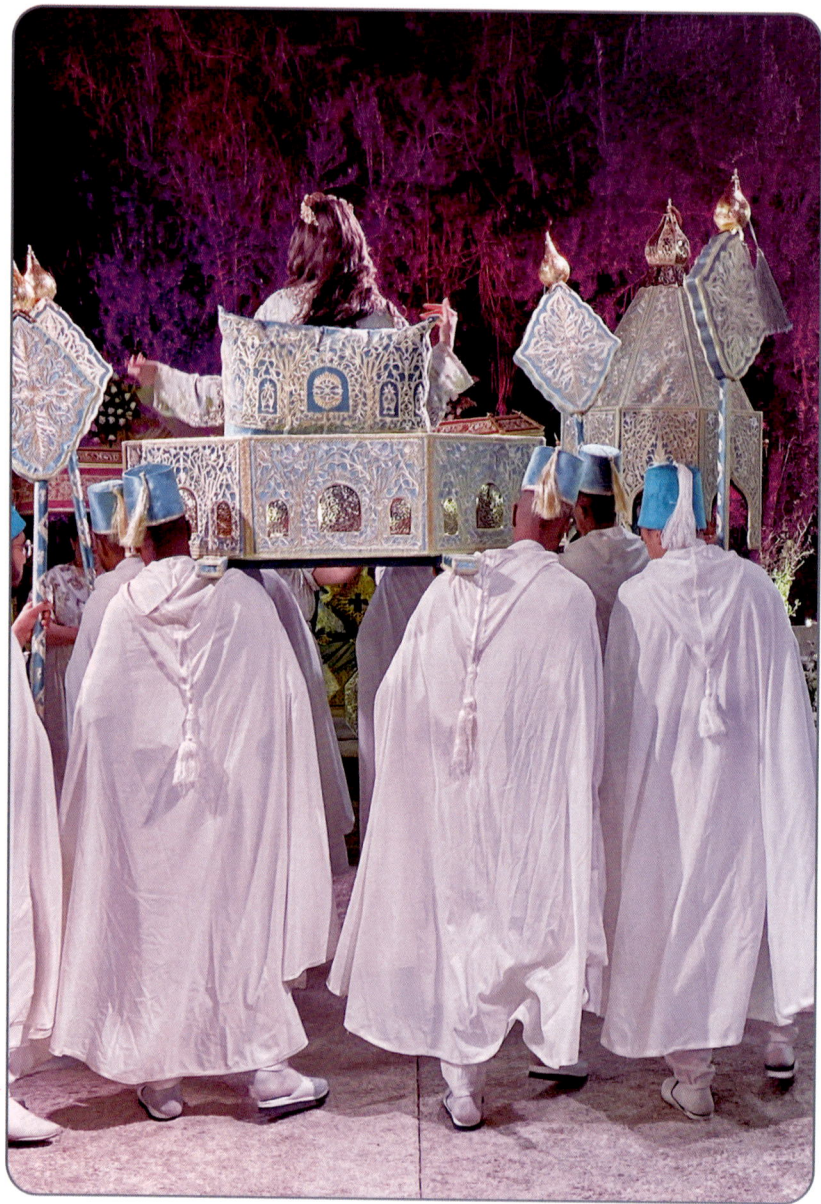

**Figure 2.4** A Common Ritual at Weddings in Morocco.

The photograph highlights the bride being carried around on the shoulders of several male bearers. Her position celebrates her place of dignity in the ceremony.

*Source.*   Photograph by Brigitte Griffith

places them below us in status. Pols (2013b) warned us about this tendency to set up certain aesthetic values that we prioritize and admire, or that essentially suit our taste. Then, we use these aesthetic or social values to organize people into differentiated classes, which engenders caste thinking and ignores merit and rights.

One of my most interesting and useful observations has been that indignities can be found in many of the social spaces that we occupy. The column ("The Knee on the Other's Neck") in Chapter 1, "Considering Race Matters," describes the event of Derek Chauvin's knee being placed on George Floyd's neck. While that column was expressly framed in the context of a racialized interaction, it is obviously relevant in any discussion of human dignity. Many friends and colleagues with whom I discussed this matter agreed that the tableau of a uniformed man firmly planting his knee on another person's vulnerable anatomy was demeaning. Floyd's status appeared to diminish before our eyes, as time passed, with a cheapening of his rank and identity. It also emphasized Chauvin's power, his control of Floyd, and his intent to inhibit Floyd's freedom. We easily recognize this type of example that characterizes indignity, and we instinctively know that we do not wish to be treated that way by any law enforcement officer or someone in authority over us.

However, we can be thankful that dignity-enhancing behavior is also visible around us, although we may at times have to be watchful to detect it. Recently, I was aboard a New York City bus that came to a stop to pick up passengers. The driver left his position up front, went a couple of rows to the back, and made some adjustments that cleared space for a motorized wheelchair. Then he opened the bus door. I could hear noises that indicated a metal floor was moving into place to accommodate the entrance of the wheelchair to the bus. Suddenly, the person in the moving chair became more clearly visible. He rolled himself to the designated open space provided by the bus driver, reversing, advancing, and backing up with the practiced elegance of an expert driver. The bus driver made sure his passenger was settled before he closed the doors and moved the bus gently forward. Not a negative word was uttered by anyone. Every bystander was patient, respectful, and considerate. Unfolding before me was a display of thoughtful caring for a fellow human being. Even the power differential between disabled and able-bodied passengers disappeared for a moment; technology was put into use during the action, patience and caring were in full view, and there seemed to be recognition that the passenger with the disability enjoyed the dignity attributed to all those who used the public transit system. The empathy and compassion extended to this unknown individual were explicitly respectful.

This manifestation of dignity in public places should remind us that dignity and indignity appear at every turn. In boyhood Barbados, the social rules undergirding dignity-enhancing behavior were present very early. I knew that from the moment I stepped out of my house, I had to be mindful of them. I could not walk past adult neighbors without saying good morning and doing so first. There was this understanding that regulated behavior. Status was linked with age. And the fundamental examples serving as immutable reference points were found in the home, at school, and in Sunday school. The village where we lived was connected to home once a child started strolling around outside. Everybody quickly appreciated who the charismatic figures in school and church were and the rank and respect attributed to them. The inherent dignity was transmitted through the culture.

Churches insisted on principles of fairness and justice that came through the elaborations of the New Testament. In a recent discussion about this claim concerning the church, a friend reminded me that sacred spaces are not always respectful of these principles. She was right, of course. Recent scandals in many different churches have verified that point. Schools relied on the British cultural principle of respect for everyone, including on the playing fields, in debates, and at scout meetings. The different systems naturally collaborated to reinforce what it meant to be a lady or a gentleman. In later years, I recognized that cultural principles are not consistently replicated in practice. One example commonly found in Caribbean culture concerns the treatment of gay individuals. Homophobia remains a significant problem and is frequently exacerbated by religious institutions.

Poverty never served as an excuse for openly disrespecting anyone. And it would be many years before I could find the courage to talk publicly and without compassion about someone. Homophobia was almost never discussed, with the now-familiar, present-day tone, by children in front of adults. The time came when that subject emerged among youngsters, coupled with mockery and quiet insults. But even then, it stayed among us and we chatted quietly. Of course, we learned curse words. But until I left Barbados as a teenager, I never heard one of my friends use an offensive term in front of his parents. My mother was blunt in her instructions. Children had to behave in public as though they had parents and upbringing. She stated it plainly: I had to behave "like I cum frum some-way." The argument was built on a foundation of personal decency, with an identity rooted in family and the Lord. In such a scheme, mothers and fathers wanted children to be proud of their family roots, their Barbadian communities, and of each other. Parents also harped on the notion that money could buy food and other necessities like a house and a bicycle for easy transportation, but not character. A friend heard me recite this explanation and quickly suggested to me that this simple, practical philosophy could not have worked for every citizen. She asked, "And what about the people in prison?" Since I lived close to that carceral institution, I humbly acknowledged the reality of her observation. Prison remains a puzzling institution in many cultures, a place where indignity is ingrained indelibly in the fabric of mundane interactions. My childhood experiences never extended in that direction, gratefully.

I return at this point to the two columns that touch on memorializing dignity in public monuments and on identity and political independence. I remind readers that Barbados was a British colony for a long time, gaining independence in 1966 and ultimately taking on the status of a republic in 2021. In a 50th anniversary speech marking the independence of Barbados, Professor Richard Drayton (2016) placed Barbados and its independence into a larger human context. Drayton described 1600s Barbados as characterized by a regime in which a few masters ruled many sub-persons. The dominant oligarchy was generally White and male, possessed land holdings, and was linked to the Anglican Church. In a sociopsychological and physical sense, the primary space was characterized by domination and not liberty. In that 50th anniversary speech, Professor Drayton (2016, p. 4) pointed out that Barbados was responsible for the Slave Code of 1661 that established a model for the "ordering and governing of Negroes." He concluded that Barbados "was a central theatre in the making of a modern world order which intertwined capitalism, racism and imperialism" (Drayton 2016, p. 4). He wished that independence would free Barbadians to experience a profound satisfaction with their country and, as well, a sense of community.

Professor Drayton's (2016) conclusion about Barbados before it gained independence was that its sociopolitical reality was characterized by poverty and injustice. There is no question that his vision of Barbados differs slightly from my boyhood notions of the island. I also lived on the outskirts of the capital city in a small village where parents could find enough for their families to eat. And so, I went to school and to church happy. It was later, when my father carried out organized migration of his family to New York City, that I realized he felt the weight of the White man's economic pressure and had no choice but to move overseas. So, the time did come when I understood what exploitation and oppression, in the context of colonial Barbados, meant in real family terms. When Drayton (2016, p. 7) suggested that being colonized meant that we would be "a perpetual child, never to be trusted to manage ourselves," I cringed. The reality of such indignity hurt deeply. This was not boyhood life. It is grasping the implications of colonization in plain daylight.

I include in this chapter's group of columns two short biographical essays of Nigerian and Black American doctors. They came from disadvantaged roots and managed themselves well, eschewing the pressure to give up struggling. They maintained their dignity in the face of impediments to easy success. I use the short narratives as reference points because they suggest hope for others. Similarly, I made clear in commenting on Justice Thomas that his argument about being ashamed to accept the offers that might come through affirmative action was cynical and limiting. Besides, he accepted other offers that came in different forms. Having no pathway out of the oppression of colonial dominance leads too readily to violence. I know that some people admire that option. But it has never found favor with me.

I underline a last reference to dignity. I refer here to the treacherous way in which the British government treated those immigrants from the Caribbean who were part of the Windrush movement. As I described it, Vanley Burke, the photographer, memorialized the presence of Blacks in British society. He photographed Black people in multiple roles: working, studying, loving, hanging out, re-creating home, worshipping, resisting, playing, getting a haircut, and debating. At the center of all the action was the quest for dignity, good health, and prosperity. In that column, I also noted that artists like the American painter Faith Ringgold and the British sculptor Thomas J. Price contributed to this exploration of value, worth, and merit among Black people.

I will return in other chapters to this theme of human dignity because of its vital and dynamic presence in the varied places that we inhabit. I have tried to describe its essence and its materiality in our daily lives. I am reminded of the British artist Lynette Yindom-Boakye whose work I saw exhibited at Yale University's Center for British Art a few years ago. I recall well the portrait, named "Amber and Jasmine" (2018), of a Black woman whose introspective pose the artist had created. She wore a headwrap and bathing suit. A curator suggested that the artist wished to focus, through fictional subjects, on humanness and gentility and to capture what the human body expresses in stillness, while seemingly being full of presence and reflection.

Edmund Pellegrino (2008) was concerned that in the context of being a patient, many of us experience a loss of identity or status. We feel, under the stress related to sickness, that our worth and dignity have been diminished. These experiences of indignity may be produced by the attitude and behavior of clinicians from any discipline as much as by the pathology that affects us. Many disorders including cancer, disfiguring pathology, and even the effects of aging may produce the experience of indignity. Gustafsson and colleagues (2013) emphasized that clinical staff, particularly in inpatient units, have an obligation to protect patients from embarrassing, humiliating, and shameful situations. And to accomplish this, nurses and doctors may be required to take extra time with certain patients and provide them extra space. The authors called this an attitude of meeting patients with dignity.

Harvey Chochinov (2007) discussed dignity-conserving care and described its fundamental elements: attitude (the establishment of empathic connections to patients), behavior (kindness and respect from clinicians), compassion (sensitivity to the patient's suffering and wanting to relieve it), and dialogue (interpersonal exchanges that verify the patient's status as a person apart from the illness). Chochinov called this the A, B, C, and D of care. He was focused on maintaining a patient's sense of worth, even as the patient worried about their loss of dignity. In fact, in these circumstances, Pellegrino (2008) suggested that some patients might believe that they were losing inherent dignity, when of course only attributed dignity was in play. Pellegrino insisted that clinicians clarify this confusion whenever they encounter it in their clinical work. Such an intervention alleviates patients' distress.

In clinical work, I have been most enamored of the ways in which human dignity may have a lasting effect on the dyadic clinician-patient relationship. Some of these effects have already been discussed in the preceding chapter that focused on race matters. In that context, the relevant mechanism was more clearly racialized discrimination. In this instance, the accent will more likely be on the differentiated value of clinician and patient. The clinician becomes somebody, and the patient is a nobody. This situation reminds me of my experiences in academic medical centers where section chiefs or department heads ostensibly conduct themselves in styles that suggest inherent superiority to those they direct. These supervisors flaunt their confidence in being above everyone within their fields of vision. They rarely smile at underlings and never offer a congratulatory word of praise about another person's success on a given project. Clinicians and executives of this sort can function effectively to some degree because they can operate purely on a knowledge base and can prescribe the correct medications and communicate instructions. On the other hand, they find it hard to connect to patients and colleagues, and they foster indignities without even realizing it. Worse, they cultivate a self-doubt in their charges that reminds me of the powerful description provided by Richard Drayton (2016, p. 7) pertaining to the psychological effects of Barbados's colonization by the British. Drayton described a self-doubt that can take over individuals and leave them feeling unable to do anything original and capable of only imitating the "special one" and seeking approval.

I hope that clinicians and administrators will recognize how dignity is fundamentally important in the clinical sphere as well as in the context of organizations, workplaces, and leisure spaces. I mentioned several artists who tried to capture dignity, to frame it in a painter's sketch, to freeze it in time and space and make it possible to touch. I mentioned efforts to memorialize dignity in public monuments and dwelt on Richard Drayton's (2016) interest in mobilizing Barbadians to mark their national independence by nurturing a feeling of profound satisfaction with their country and encouraging whole communities to have self-confidence.

Indignity has been present in political discourse over the last decade or so in the United States in a novel form. I never expected that competing politicians would mention someone's hairstyle or manner of speaking with an intent to dehumanize or debase the other. Despite its presence all around us, it seems hard for some to grasp how noxious the experience of repeated indignities can be.

## Questions to Ponder

1. Can you define the two common types of human dignity and give illustrative examples?
2. Can you describe several examples of indignities endured by patients on a hospital ward?
3. Should we spend any time trying to think about the authors of violence as capable of seeing dignity in others?
4. When you travel that imaginary road and arrive at the fork, do you ever contemplate the road not taken? Is it worth the effort?
5. Do you enjoy the experience of attributing dignity to others? Or is trusting in intrinsic dignity enough for you?

## References

Adshead G, Horne E: The Devil You Know: Stories of Human Cruelty and Compassion. New York, Scribner, 2021

Brooks P: Narrative transactions—does the law need a narratology? Yale J Law Humanit 18(1):1–28, 2006

Chawla D: Tracing home's habits: affective rhythms, in Stories of Home: Place, Identity, Exile. Edited by Chawla D, Jones SH. New York, Lexington Books, 2015, pp 3–15

Chochinov HM: Dignity and the essence of medicine: the A, B, C, and D of dignity conserving care. BMJ 335(7612):184–187, 2007 17656543

Desai MU: Travel as qualitative method: travel in psychology's history and in Medard Boss' Sojourn to India. J Humanist Psychol 54:494–507, 2014

Drayton R: The Time of Sovereignty: The History of Political Independence and Its Future. Presented as the Sir Winston Scott Memorial Lecture, Central Bank of Barbados, November 28, 2016. Available at: https://www.centralbank.org.bb/viewPDF/documents/2021-12-27-05-07-25-Transcript-of-41st-SWSML---Dr.-Richard-Drayton.pdf. Accessed June 15, 2024.

Drayton R: Barbados: the long road to the republic. Stabroek News, November 29, 2021

Gastambide DJ: A People's History of Psychoanalysis. New York, Lexington Books, 2019

Gustafsson LK, Wigerblad A, Lindwall L: Respecting dignity in forensic care: the challenge faced by nurses of maintaining patient dignity in clinical caring situations. J Psychiatr Ment Health Nurs 20(1):1–8, 2013 22417206

Hackim D, Becker J: The long crusade of Clarence and Ginni Thomas. New York Times Magazine, February 22, 2018

Hickling F: Decolonization of Psychiatry in Jamaica. New York, Springer, 2021

Moss D: On having whiteness. J Am Psychoanal Assoc 69(2):355–371, 2021

Norko MA: What is truth? The spiritual quest of forensic psychiatry. J Am Acad Psychiatry Law 46(1):10–22, 2018 29618531

Pellegrino P: The lived experience of human dignity, in Human Dignity and Bioethics: Essays Commissioned by the President's Council on Bioethics. Washington, DC, President's Council on Bioethics, 2008, pp 513–539

Petrusich A: The otherworldly compositions of an Ethiopian nun. New Yorker, April 17, 2023

Pols J: Washing the patient: dignity and aesthetic values in nursing care. Nurs Philos 14(3):186–200, 2013a

Pols J: Through the looking glass: good looks and dignity in care. Med Health Care Philos 16(4):953–966, 2013b

Sulmasy DP: The varieties of human dignity: a logical and conceptual analysis. Med Health Care Philos 16(4):937–944, 2013

Walcott D: The Prodigal. New York, Farrar, Straus & Giroux, 2004

# 3

# Facing Disability

# Columns From *Psychiatric News*

## The Silence of the Deaf[1]

Several decades have gone by since that morning when I passed him the ball. He ran into a forward position from the left wing, but diagonally, and stretched out his left arm at a slight upward slant so I could see it. Neither of us wanted to attract attention from the opposing team. He couldn't verbally ask for the ball anyway, as he couldn't speak. I didn't say anything because he couldn't hear. As he turned to straighten his position toward the goal, I kicked the ball to his right with what soccer aficionados call a perfectly weighted pass. The ball went by him with its initial speed. As he moved more quickly, and the ball slowed down, he was on track to connect with it in about 10 yards. He reached it and shot it into the net in a one-touch move. What a beauty! After the game, he came toward me. Five yards away, he stopped, clasping both hands at chest level with palms touching each other. He bowed with a grin that said thanks, and I returned the gesture. For a single special moment, I had entered the silent world of the deaf.

That distant memory came back to me as I entered the Pantheon in Paris this summer to visit the exposition "L'Histoire Silencieuse des Sourds" ("The Silent History of the Deaf"). The displays recounted a brief history of the deaf in France with occasional allusions to what had taken place in the United States. At first, I found "silent" in the title puzzling. However, as I proceeded with the visit, things got clearer. In some cases, a child's deafness is picked up very late by the family, and the youngster never develops speech and other communication skills. Thus, the child remains isolated in a uniquely silent community. I've also noticed how some older folk, losing their capacity to hear, avoid seeking medical help to adapt to the incipient disability. The result is progressive isolation in an environment of decreasing social interaction and increasing silence. The exposition's title also invites reflection on the world of silence inhabited by many of those suffering from severe mental and other chronic illnesses and those in extreme environments such as the segregated units of prisons. At first, the retreat may be comforting. But soon, the deterioration of important social and cognitive skills becomes a problem.

---

[1] Adapted with permission from Griffith EEH: The Silence of the Deaf. *Psychiatric News*, October 2019. Copyright © 2019 American Psychiatric Association. All rights reserved.

The exposition shone a light on my ignorance. I was not fluent in the theoretical connections between the sign language used by the deaf and mechanisms developed by monks of the Middle Ages who lived in silence. I was embarrassed that as a forensic psychiatrist I had never heard of the late–18th century French case of Madeleine Le Mansois (1750–1826). At the time, she appealed to the highest court in the land to overturn a lower court ruling that had stopped her from marrying the man of her choice because of her disability. She won the case, aiding in the development of the concept of "free consent" regarding matrimony, so long as a woman could make her preference clear. At least I had heard of the advocacy movement that the exposition had termed "deaf militancy." The movement focused on a language for the deaf that would help them acquire skills for social, intellectual, and cultural situations.

I have spent a substantial part of my professional life fighting on behalf of disadvantaged groups. But, partly because of their small numbers in the system, a fraction of that time has involved representation of those who cannot hear. I recalled how difficult it had been for me to obtain optimal psychiatric care for several hospitalized patients with severe hearing impairment. I had to represent their needs formally to the administration and insist that outside experts be hired to carry out specialized assessments and provide care. In my experience, many caregivers lack the requisite training. Few of my colleagues have mastered the art of signing and immersed themselves in the culture of the deaf.

I shall remember the scene at the Pantheon's exposition. Individuals with hearing impairments were well represented, visible by their vigorous signing to each other, obviously discussing the salient points of each presentation. Their relaxed appearance said that they felt they belonged there—and indeed they did. They were signifying and celebrating, proud that curators wanted to feature historic contributions to the culture of the deaf.

## Reply to Larry Davidson on Recovery[2]

The Yale professor Larry Davidson (2018) published a thoughtful commentary with the interrogative title: "Is There a Future for Recovery?" Curiosity got the better of me for two reasons: First, he and his colleagues

---

[2] Adapted with permission from Griffith EEH: Reply to Larry Davidson on Recovery. *Psychiatric News*, March 2020. Copyright © 2020 American Psychiatric Association. All rights reserved.

at the Yale School of Medicine are among the major theorists in the country discussing the recovery movement in mental health. Second, he and his senior collaborator, Professor Michael Rowe, have long been responsible for tutoring me about recovery.

Davidson noted that Patricia Deegan's seminal article (1988) ("Recovery: The Lived Experience of Rehabilitation") described the concept of recovery as people's life experience of confronting and overcoming the challenges of a disability. Recovery also provides renewal of one's self and purpose in relation to the potential limiting effects of the disability. Davidson remarked that the conceptualization of recovery coincided with the eventual inclusion of psychiatric disability in the 1990 Americans With Disabilities Act. He was originally pleased with this linkage of serious mental illnesses to what he called a disability-rights framework. He agreed that this approach brought change in mental health policy and practice and in the expectations of those suffering from mental illness. However, he worried that the disability framework may be on the wane.

Davidson mentioned concrete achievements, though, such as increased emphasis on community care; supports for care centered on housing, employment, and education; and development of self-help tools. So why had he become worried? He explained that his first concern was linked to the de-emphasis of the disability in the definition of recovery. In other words, recovery is now seen by some as a unique or deeply personal journey. Thus, caregivers de-emphasized acute medical care; in some quarters, hospitals were considered less prominent and even useless.

Davidson's second major concern was what he described as "neglect of the social and cultural determinants of mental health" (Davidson 2018, p. 12). Some of us have long noted this problem, simply because some patients were being discharged from hospitals with little regard for their poverty, social standing, and even their complex medical status apart from their mental illness. This occurred in the face of clinical understanding that serious mental illness and significant physical illness compounded by structural factors like poverty or racism can be devastating for anyone.

I understand Davidson's worrying, especially as he is a good friend and colleague. He has also worked hard on behalf of severely ill patients. From time to time, I have been disappointed by those who have distorted the principles that he and his colleagues set up to guide the implementation of recovery theory. For example, there was a time when U.S. Department of Justice representatives visited hospitals around the country, preaching recovery for all and ignoring the heterogeneity in outcomes produced by the mental illness disability. They also seemed unaware that state hospitals were providing care for seriously ill patients, those for whom clinical recovery was often most difficult. None of this was Davidson's fault, of course.

His article ended on an important point, as he looked to the future. He focused on the group of individuals with "prolonged disabilities ... who do not recover in the conventional, clinical sense of the term" (Davidson 2018, p. 12). These individuals have a hard time living with their illnesses, struggle mightily with their psychosocial disabilities, and confront varying forms of isolation and exclusion from their communities. Davidson wants them "let in" as they are (i.e., disabled) to the general community around them without having to "fit in" by hiding their disabilities. Davidson made clear that this is a major challenge for the future, and he is, of course, right. Clinical recovery for this group is not a casual challenge. It demands concentrated attention, creativity, futuristic imagination, and a commitment to humanity from a collective of clinicians, politicians, policy leaders, and academics. We should develop a new approach to their care and to preserving their dignity.

## Creative Writing and Psychiatric Rehabilitation[3]

These days it feels like a blessing to receive some positive news in my email inbox. This time it arrived in a message from Fellowship Place, a health care agency created well over 50 years ago. It has been serving adults living with mental illness in the Greater New Haven area of Connecticut. Fellowship, as many in the mental health community call it affectionately, is widely known for offering rehabilitation services that include supportive housing, vocational training, and homeless engagement. The objective is wellness, independence, and meaningful living. There are also programs that promote creative expression through painting, writing, and music. The email message contained the winter 2021 issue of *The Beacon*, Fellowship's literary journal.

---

[3] Adapted with permission from Griffith EEH: Creative Writing and Psychiatric Rehabilitation. *Psychiatric News*, April 2021. Copyright © 2021 American Psychiatric Association. All rights reserved.

Quotations from students' writings in *The Beacon* are used with permission of Fellowship Place.

Perusing the 10 pages of text brought back the pleasure I took in writing "Visibility in a Psychiatric Hospital's Museum" (Griffith 2019). That column was an account of my visit to a painting exposition at Paris's Sainte-Anne Psychiatric Hospital. The creative work had been done by individuals receiving care at the hospital. I remember thinking about the role of the visual arts in our treatment plans and the cost in human and financial resources, institutional commitment, building space, and the technical expertise of teachers.

*The Beacon* is a wonderful example of what the engagement in writing can produce. About 14 individuals took part in this edition of the journal, which encompassed both poetry and short essays. Both forms of writing recounted personal experiences of times gone by and recollections of encounters with places and people. One prose piece talked of breeding a new, enormous vegetable from the cabbage family. Another author contemplated outer space as the last genealogical frontier. On the very first page of the journal, there was a note mentioning that some of the contributions were written while members of the group were confined during the coronavirus disease 2019 (COVID-19) pandemic. One writer mused about lessons learned from 2020, such as the acquisition of inner peace. Notice was taken of some similarity between the confinement and the movie story of Anne Frank. Someone regretted that COVID-19 had caused suspension of a theater group's meetings, which resulted in a feeling of disrupted friendship. The loss was partly diminished by a cat's companionship.

I wondered whether one of the writing group's exercises may have focused on personal identity, as several poets addressed the subject.

> Who do I want to be?
> I want to be a high school graduate.
> I want to be a Christian author.
> I want to be a loving wife, mother and friend.

One writer was more contemplative:

> Sometimes I am confused.
> Sometimes I am confident.
> Most of the time, I am love.
> This is me too.

Another invoked a sense of freedom:

> Who do I want to be?
> I want to be free.
> I want to be at peace.
> I want to be awake.
> This is who I am.
> This is who I want to be.

This poet seemed focused on the goings-on within the environment.

I enjoyed reading the writing quietly, then reciting the language out loud, and finding myself transported by my soliloquy. The words took on life, and I could feel the writers' reflection and imagination at work. In my reading, I grasped why experts like Deborah Philips, Liz Linington, and Debra Penman (1999) recommended creative writing's place in mental health therapeutics and rehabilitation. It facilitates the expression and management of memories, while also promoting trust and community. There is a positive effect on concentration and orientation. People who write note their enhanced sensitivity to others and awareness of their surroundings. This comes through practiced observation and imagination, as expressed in *The Beacon*.

> While basking in the warmth of a drowsy, blazing, hot sun,
> Friendly, furry, brown squirrels play, jump and run,
> Mating, multiplying, take a husband or wife,
> Eating acorns, and nuts,
> Surviving,
> Grasping hold of life,
> Swiftly climbing green leafy oak trees,
> Inhaling fresh air from a summer breeze,
> As colorful rainbows light up the sky with their smile,
> In their own language, squirrels sing the love song of the wild.

## 'Homes' at the Sainte-Anne Hospital Museum[4]

I wrote before, in late 2019, about the Musée d'Art et d'Histoire de l'Hôpital Sainte-Anne, known popularly as the MAHHSA. It is a landmark in Paris and an iconic structure among psychiatric hospitals

---

[4] Adapted with permission from Griffith EEH: 'Homes' at the Sainte-Anne Hospital Museum. *Psychiatric News*, May 2022. Copyright © 2022 American Psychiatric Association. All rights reserved.

worldwide. I could not ignore its present exposition, "Maisons" ("Homes"), which I visited earlier this year. I take responsibility for my translation of the title/theme, recognizing that the French word could be considered as "houses" or "homes." MAHHSA's own description of the exposition convinced me that *homes* is the better term.

The *Guide d'Exposition* maintained that the collection would evoke a variety of personal images and ideological and architectural conceptualizations of lifestyles. The exhibition would also facilitate metaphorical and imaginary projections about the unreal and the concrete, as well as of true and false memories supported by sensory and bodily experiences. The exposition, divided into four sections, was based on close to 110 works from the museum's collection and a dozen other additions from contemporary artists.

"La Maison-Hôpital (Home-Hospital)" was the first part of the collection. The guide's commentary acknowledged that the old term of *asylum* implied a place of constraint and confinement. In this section of the exhibition, artists depicted a familiar place of residence, signifying that the hospital had evolved into a place of ritualized daily living. Having spent decades discussing the meaning of the psychiatric hospital, I know this recognition of the hospital as home for some people suffering with psychiatric illness distresses many theorists. Nonetheless, it remains reality and deserves memorializing by artists.

An untitled 1906 charcoal drawing by H.A.R., one of the earliest artists in the Sainte-Anne collection, is shown in Figure 3.1. In this work, she illustrates women performing the domestic task of sewing. It is hard to determine everyone's degree of commitment to the activity. However, we know the significance of structured activity in the psychiatric hospital and possibilities of community within a small group. The women's attire and aesthetics suggest fellowship and dignity. Experts think that the artist was formally trained, with experience in the use of charcoal and sanguine crayons. Her work bears witness to the rehabilitation activity found in psychiatric hospitals at the beginning of the 1900s.

"Vers La Demeure (Towards the Residence)," the 2nd section, marks the movement to becoming sedentary, taking up residence, and suspending time. The artists in this group are said to raise questions about the function of the residential space. They provide different notions of the size and location of the house and its integration into the surrounding scenery.

In the 3rd section, "A l'Intérieur de l'Intime (Inside the Intimate)," I felt I was inside more private and intimate spaces. As the formal

*Facing Disability*

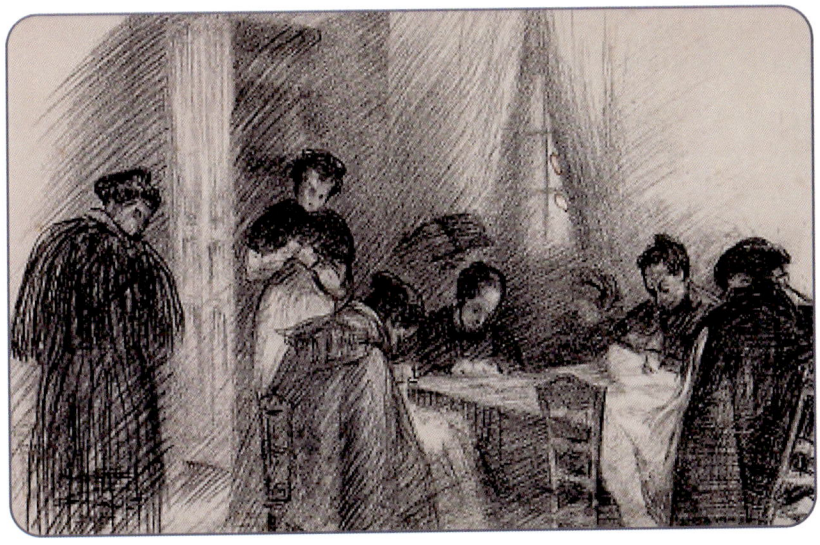

**Figure 3.1** Untitled, 1906, by H.A.R.

Drawing of women sewing; charcoal on paper.

*Source.* Copyright © CEE MAHHSA, Musée d'Art et d'Histoire de l'Hôpital Sainte-Anne, Paris, Copyright © Dominique Baliko.

museum description stated, these paintings represented a variety of activities that symbolized rest, leisure, and even boredom. Intimacy was also reflected in special family spaces or a particular kind of domestic activity. The untitled 1950 crayon-and-gouache work by René Héroult in Figure 3.2 represents the intimate space of a visual artist. The tools of the craft are present, with a work in progress at the center of the painting. We are left to wonder about the solitary cat as companion. Even so, the colors evoke a certain warmth and vibrance.

The 4th section, "Rêve d'Habitation (Dream of Home Space)," represents for me the most creative and unexpected contributions to the exposition. The artists constructed their dream of a place to live. The guide booklet drew attention to the tall towers, enormous castles, utopian towns, and presence of machines, while pointing out that some of these imagined spaces seemed uninhabitable.

Leaving the art exhibition, I treasured the experience offered by this unique collection. Sainte-Anne compelled me to mull over what I had just seen. I wanted to know more about the artists and their thoughts about Sainte-Anne. Had it been more a place of healthful restoration than a zone of banishment and invisibility? Had they made a

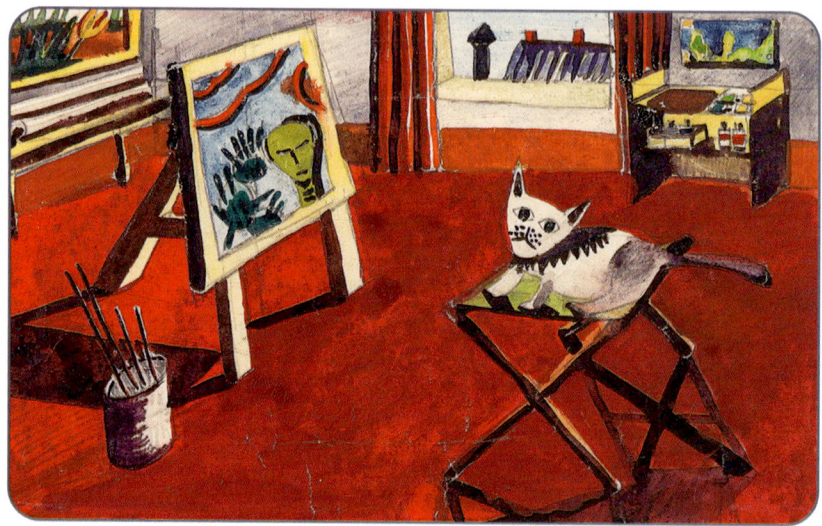

**Figure 3.2** Untitled, 1950, by René Héroult.

The intimate space of a visual artist; crayon and gouache. The tools of the craft are present in the painting, with a work in progress at the center and a solitary cat as companion.

*Source.* Copyright © CEE MAHHSA, Musée d'Art et d'Histoire de l'Hôpital Sainte-Anne, Paris, Copyright © Dominique Baliko.

solid connection between place and health? Finally, did their creativity afford them a sense of freedom that conferred dignity and enhanced their well-being? I hope so. There is certainly no doubt that this psychiatric hospital museum is catalyzing thought about its patients' humanity and our duty to interrogate ourselves about how we interact with them.

## Memories of a Community Hospital[5]

In 1974, I was introduced to Dr. Gabriel Koz (Figure 3.3). He had been director of the Department of Psychiatry at New York City's Lincoln Hospital since November 1969. When we met, I was a first-year resident in psychiatry, unsure of the department's history and ignorant of Dr.

---

[5] Adapted with permission from Griffith EEH: Memories of a Community Hospital. *Psychiatric News*, July 2022. Copyright © 2022 American Psychiatric Association. All rights reserved.

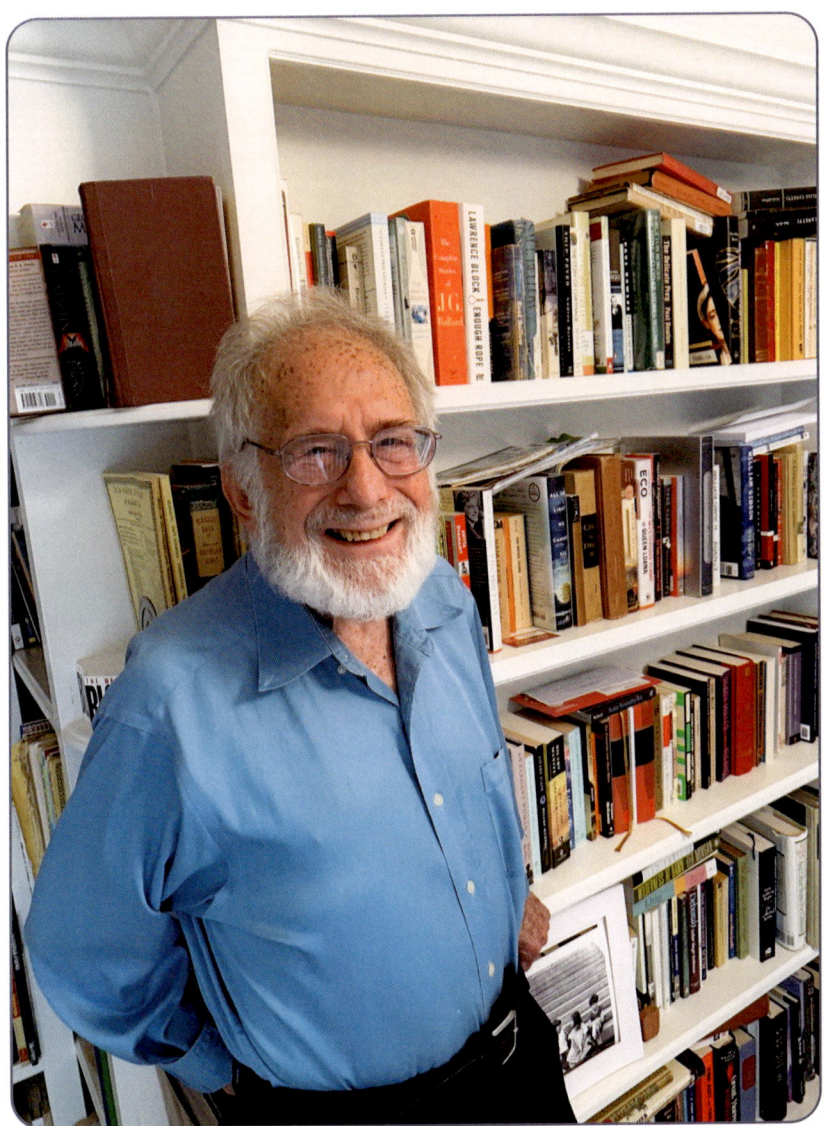

**Figure 3.3**  Gabriel Koz, M.D.

He brought unity to the Department of Psychiatry at Lincoln Hospital in the Bronx, New York, at a time of civil unrest and social upheaval. Following that, he served as medical director of Eastern State Hospital in Williamsburg, Virginia. He died in 2024.

*Source.*   Photograph by Daniel Koz.

Koz's place in it. When I finished training in 1977, I went off to join the faculty at Yale. Dr. Koz left the same year to head the Manhattan Psychiatric Center, a major facility in New York State's constellation of psychiatric hospitals. After his distinctive and successful stint at Lincoln, he was known in the arena of psychiatric hospital administration. We lost contact for decades and then reestablished our connection in 2005 at a lecture he delivered on receiving the Administrative Psychiatry Award from the American Psychiatric Association (APA). Our common Lincoln experience certainly gave us much to discuss. At the top of the list were our memories of the hospital and what we had learned from our stay in the famous New York City neighborhood known as the South Bronx. That community was the place to reflect on the intersection of mental illness and psychosocial factors of all sorts, as well as the need for specially sensitive and thoughtful caregivers.

In this predominantly Latino and Black neighborhood, I was studying psychiatry while observing the intersection of class, race, and poverty. I was an immigrant from Barbados. Dr. Koz had arrived at Lincoln from South Africa by way of London and Boston, two cities where he had done his psychiatry training. He had also spent time in Israel, and I had lived in France. We brought an international perspective to the struggles all around us. His medical degree was from the University of the Witwatersrand in South Africa. My medical education had taken place at the University of Strasbourg in France. We had come to know each other in the South Bronx at a time when community psychiatry was enjoying remarkable popularity. The late 1960s, of course, was the era of civil rights militancy. The mood was spreading to related domains of health, education, justice, housing, and transportation.

Dr. Koz (2021) memorialized his years at Lincoln, as well as his life story, in his autobiography. He explained that Lincoln Hospital had an 1839 start somewhere in Manhattan, occupying several locations before moving to the South Bronx in 1899. In November 1963, the New York City Health and Hospitals Corporation contracted with the Albert Einstein College of Medicine to provide mental health services at Lincoln Hospital. Coalitions of medical schools and public hospitals were regularly created to upgrade medical services delivered to communities, especially the disadvantaged ones. The White professionals assigned to Lincoln by Einstein gradually encountered significant opposition from Black and Latino staff and community activists. Buoyed by the national civil rights protests in progress, the local militants demanded greater community influence and even control of health care services. A major strike occurred in March 1969, and an unsettling result of these conditions was repeated changes in the leadership of Lincoln's Department of Psychiatry. In his narrative, Dr. Koz noted the psychiatry program was in chaos and near collapse when he arrived as the new director in November of that year. The community was rife with disorderliness, as well as discontent.

S. R. Kaplan and M. Roman (1973) described these events in *The Organization and Delivery of Mental Health Services in the Ghetto: The Lincoln Hospital Experience*. The events at Lincoln had become a case history for study by community psychiatrists, administrators, and politicians in the United States. In a subsequent review of the book in *Psychiatric Services*, Dr. Lucy Ozarin (1974) stated that Black and Puerto Rican groups were vying for power in the community. In a different assessment, Claudewell Thomas (1974) noted that the university system's major preoccupation was giving accolades to its faculty, while other staff received little recognition and were left in dreariness. Opinions about what had transpired at Lincoln were legion. Dr. Koz's role was to provide steady leadership and build community among the partisan stakeholders.

In his narrative, Dr. Koz confronted the tensions and problems he had faced at Lincoln with a certain equanimity. He recognized the restlessness of a divided community, fueled by the clash of ethnicities; the anti–Vietnam War sentiments; the presence of civil rights furor; neighborhood crime; rampant substance use; and poverty. There were also the structural dilemmas provoked and exacerbated by several bureaucracies: city, state, and federal in addition to university and medical school. Nevertheless, his tenure at Lincoln Hospital had been exciting, and he had stabilized the department. Lincoln was a symbol of context's place in confronting psychiatric disability.

I, too, left Lincoln with indelible memories. It was there that I first met and heard Chester Pierce deliver a lecture. The Saturday evening when a staff member took me to a séance of Puerto Rican Espiritismo remains a highlight of my excursions into psychiatry and religion. These memories remain next to my mind's photograph of Gabriel Koz moving among the major cultures in the South Bronx displaying remarkable flexibility and dignity and representing reconciliation.

## Seeing the World Through Writers' Eyes[6]

Almost 2 years ago, I wrote a column, which appears earlier in this chapter, on psychiatric rehabilitation and creative writing (2021). It highlighted a program run by Fellowship Place, a health care agency serving adults and located in the Greater New Haven area of Connecticut. Their mission, as I said then, was wellness, independence, and meaningful living. Among their programs were those that promoted creative expression through painting, writing, and music. I was attracted once again to Fellowship's literary journal, *The Beacon*, as I eyed the summer 2022 edition, wondering what the program's writers were doing presently.

The new issue reaffirms, in an invitation printed on the last page, that Fellowship's Writers Group "is a safe space for writers from all genres and levels of experience to come together and share their work." The reaffirmation was so simply stated and meaningful! I wondered whether it would garner more attention if placed on the front page. In nine pages of text, 15 individuals produced a variety of writing forms: poetry, essays, and journalistic reports.

One identifiable theme of this edition was summertime. Tim S. wrote of events from his youth: the visit of an ice cream truck to his neighborhood and a trip with his parents to see the Yankees play baseball in New York City. Schnaider T., describing a perfect summer day, could "hear the birds chirping and singing all types of melodies," while the squirrels ran after each other and jumped in the air. Julie N. talked of creating a new holiday for her part of the country. Celebrants of the event would wear some sort of Mardi Gras costume. On rethinking, she allowed people to show up dressed as a teardrop, a wallflower, a unicorn, or anything else. There were perceptible elements of grace, freedom, and movement in these writers' visions.

I enjoy an author's invitation to view an imaginary landscape while framing the story. On page 5 of this issue, Nicole K. and Desiree B. penned vignettes on the subject of "My Spirit Animal." Nicole imagined being a lioness: eating a lot, hunting for food, swimming, fighting with siblings, and exploring the environment. Desiree admired the

---

[6] Adapted with permission from Griffith EEH: Seeing the World Through Writers' Eyes. *Psychiatric News*, November 2022. Copyright © 2022 American Psychiatric Association. All rights reserved.

Quotations from and descriptions and representations of students' writings in *The Beacon* are used with permission of Fellowship Place.

beauty, grace, and delicacy of a monarch butterfly, sitting on flower petals and smelling their sweet fragrance. Connections between us and the fauna we encounter domestically and through films and our imagination continue to amaze me. We invest them with our hopes, love, dreams, and sometimes our deepest fears.

There was also playfulness in the writing. On page 7, Nichole D. described the world waking up to the color yellow as the Beatles sang "Here Comes the Sun" and people recognized there was no ongoing war. Yolanda W. conceptualized a world seen in different shades of red. Attracted by its power, she framed the trees, grass, and flowers in dark red, fitted against a sky bathed in pink and purple, and a ground painted violet. I could not decide what my favorite color is, and I did not dare to imagine a uni-shaded universe. I have seen vast impressive fields of yellow sunflowers on trips to Europe and been spellbound by the variegated canvases of southern European and Caribbean artists. The painting by Jacques Richard Chéry, a 20th-century Haitian artist, illustrates this combination of humor intermingled with bright colors (Figure 3.4). The result is a landscape of optimism and joy amid mundane country life.

Lynda S. composed a short autobiographical essay on her proudest moment, "the design and creation of 12 stained glass windows for a Jewish temple." She said proudly, "I designed the themed window from the Rabbi's desires for his temple." And the pride encompassed her family. "My family came down … for one installation and dedication ceremony. I'll never forget the words my dad said to me. …That had been the first time he ever said that he was proud of me." I have recently been reading about the differences between intrinsic and extrinsic or attributed dignity. Many of us hear repeatedly about our inherent, inviolable dignity. We still long for social dignity, the dignity attributed by groups and people who are important to us. Parents play an important role in this ritual of attribution.

I could not contain my curiosity about these writers and their personal worlds. Disentangling their writing processes from the themes they elaborated and the memories they evoked was complex and delicate. I liked their plainly spoken observations and the humanizing of traits found in life around them. Rereading their writing made me think of Anton Hart's (2017) notions of radical openness and curiosity. The more genuinely curious I became, the more my connection to these writers grew.

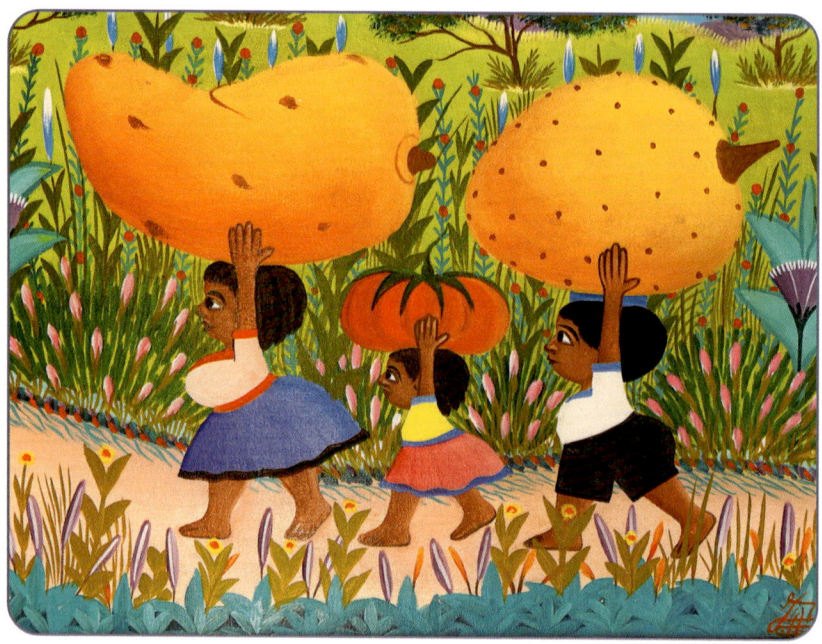

**Figure 3.4** Three Children With Fruit by Jacques Richard Chéry.

Chéry, a 20th-century Haitian artist, is known for his humorous scenes of life and use of bright colors.

*Source.*   Private Anonymous Collection. Used with permission.

# End-of-Year Rituals and New Year Promises[7]

I have always liked public and private rituals that mark the transition from one calendar year to another. In these moments of ceremony, I like to reflect on my trespasses and transgressions. If some humility sets in, I acknowledge having fallen short. With the arrival of the new year, a secular advent season arrives, and I formulate promises for the future and a new beginning of sorts. It may be a good time to change bad habits and start afresh with hope and a commitment to treat others with more grace and compassion. In my case, the events

---

[7] Adapted with permission from Griffith EEH: End-of-Year Rituals and New Year Promises. *Psychiatric News,* March 2024. Copyright © 2024 American Psychiatric Association. All rights reserved.

that mark interyear transitions have often been connected to religious rituals such as the traditional church services held on December 24 and 31. The former fostered a sense of community through the singing of hymns and carols we all knew by heart. As for the latter, what we called the *watch-night* service, old-timers loved bragging to friends about having witnessed timepieces move past midnight. "Last night I watched the New Year come in, man. You should have heard those tenors at All Souls Church." Mentioning the singing or the sermon verified the claim's truth and deepened its solemn character. Of course, that did not always guarantee faithful execution of full-throated New Year promises.

One should expect that end-of-year happenings come in a variety of forms. I have friends who look forward to attending the December 31 performance by the Alvin Ailey dance troupe in New York City. They have regaled me with descriptions of Ailey's fabulous creation called "Revelations," in which popular gospel songs sung live, like "Wade in the Water" and "Fix Me, Jesus," serve as background to the modern dance piece featuring delightful costumes. Other friends prefer a simple dinner and amicable conversation about the ebbing old year and hopes about the one to come. These examples of culture-bound gatherings seem to magically promote togetherness and introspection.

I recognize that end-of-year time is not, for everyone, a leisurely stroll in a rose garden. I am also aware that ridding oneself of old habits and acquiring new ones require courage. Besides, there are other elements in play that are beyond our control. In addition, some of us define the end-of-year concept differently. Teachers and students may see the school year as the important reference point. Others go by the fiscal year. Romantic souls think only of the anniversary of their first encounter with a lover. And a friend of mine measures everything by the day and month of his ordination to the priesthood.

Last December 18, I attended the Forty-Year Celebration of the Yale Cellos, an ensemble of about a dozen cellists under the direction of a faculty conductor. Members of the group change annually, as they are graduate student performers. I had previously heard them play on several occasions, and I enjoyed their rich harmonic sound. I looked forward to using the occasion as an end-of-year ritual and to hide from the ordinary reminders of violence, brutal suffering, plain injustice, and uncontrollable events like earthquakes and tsunamis.

The evening's program started with Richard Wagner's "Feierliches Stück," excerpted from his three-act 1850 Romantic opera, "Lohengrin." This opening piece was performed by a quartet from the larger group.

The music was a beautiful rendering of a solemn lament that set the stage for me to drift into reconsidering my year's experiences. The second and fourth pieces on the program, Franz Joseph Haydn's "Cello Concerto No. 2 in D Major" and his "Cello Concerto No. 1 in C Major," were arranged by Douglas Moore. Haydn (1732–1809) composed the No. 1 in the 1760s and completed the second about 20 years later. The two concerti offered the audience opportunities to sample different stylistic expressions of a solo cello performance. The dynamic, aggressive, quick sections reminded me of the traditional court music and dance of the time. The "Elegy" of Dave Brubeck (1920–2012), whose jazz arrangements I listened to in college, was performed between the two Haydn works. Brubeck's opus was a sad tone poem of sublime chords. The soloist in this piece offered a love message full of regret and peaceful longing. It made me curious about what had given birth to such creativity. The music effectively accompanied my thoughts.

I am not courageous enough to detail the stories that came to mind as I sat through the concert. Neither will I report dramatically of having refashioned my life. But I can say confidently that the concert was an example of my using a cultural habit to soothe myself and evaluate some things. We should seek an equivalent routine that fits us for this purpose. Then we can search out landscapes, two at the most, from among the several that characterize our daily life rhythms. I refer to the ones we can feel in the spaces we occupy from one day to the next. Common examples are the home space, work/school space, social/leisure space, personal health space, and the sacred space. Choosing two spaces is enough for one end-of-year season. Leave the rest to another: Lent, Easter, or the summer, if you operate in terms of seasons or climate. And, if possible, seek a partner to join in the adventure. That way, you can talk over the approach, the sense of solitude or failure, and how good it feels to think about caring for self and someone else.

## Reflecting on Forgiveness[8]

I have been participating recently in a weekly group discussion with psychoanalysts. The talk generally focuses on scholarly writings of analysts, and sometimes others, who have been reflecting on race and

---

[8] Adapted with permission from Griffith EEH: Reflecting on Forgiveness. *Psychiatric News*, April 2024. Copyright © 2024 American Psychiatric Association. All rights reserved.

its place in analytic discourse. I am indebted to this group's interest in and disciplined exploration of this intriguing arena of scholarship and clinical practice. In my case, it has meant expanding my intellectual horizons and engaging with a literature that, without explicit encouragement, I would probably have left untouched.

Not long ago, the assigned reading was Chapter 12 ("After the Offense: Thoughts on Forgiveness") from Donald Moss's (2017) text *At War With the Obvious: Disruptive Thinking in Psychoanalysis* (Routledge). Moss is a well-known public intellectual who enjoys linking psychoanalysis to contemporary social and political problems. Our group selected this chapter for exploration because it focused on forgiveness, a theme we have encountered repeatedly in texts framing discrimination, caste, and privilege.

In the chapter's introduction, Moss asserts that in the relation between any two people, "along with questions of retaliation, revenge, and punishment, the question of forgiveness emerges" (Moss 2017, p. 153). He suggests that our ignorance of the term *forgiveness* stems from its lack of structured meaning, as well as from a plethora of interpretations that we attribute to it. Moss uses the film *Facing Fear* (Cohen 2014) to help explain his frustration with our tendency to use terms, inexact as they are, to communicate the fundamental principles by which many of us live. The film's narrative portrays a young gay man's urban encounter with a group of skinheads. They get into a fight with the youth and mercilessly beat him almost to death while taunting him.

Twenty years later, one of the skinheads and the victim of the attack realize that they are both working in the same museum. They eventually get past the chasm that separates them and start "working together, giving presentations on forgiveness" (Moss 2017, p. 154). Moss comments that the short film "celebrates forgiveness without going into its workings" (Moss 2017, p. 154). The film leans on and confirms the idea that this sort of forgiveness is "best treated at its face value of self-evident good" (Moss 2017, p. 154). Our psychoanalyst-author is not pleased with this reflexive conventional outcome. He wants contemplation of a more balanced story that includes consideration of the gay man eschewing forgiveness and even planning some form of revenge. Moss proposes that the victim should be no more "obligated to forgive than he is to seek vengeance" (Moss 2017, p. 154). He dismisses, somewhat casually, the notion that forgiveness should be seen as the film's hero, while revenge is sort of banished offscreen. He is similarly not pleased with the easy slide from forgiveness into strategic reconciliation, while vengeance is relegated ignominiously. Moss states that impulsive forgiveness or vengeance, while promising relief, is not the way of psychoanalysis. After the offense, there must be a pause that heralds the transformation of impulsive thinking, which is, I believe, his gift to us.

Not surprisingly at all, Donald Moss employs case vignettes to be more persuasive. In doing so, he lapses into a specialized style of narrative that requires of us a disciplined familiarity with clinical praxis. However, at the end of his reflections, he concludes that the important goal for clinician and patient is "construction of a zone safe enough to promote separateness and thought" (Moss 2017, p. 160). He underlines it. The essential task is for the patient "to find an exit from the … zone of pure reflex" (Moss 2017, p. 160). Then will come nonreflexive possibilities for forgiveness and revenge.

It seems to me an overly intellectualized demand. I thought psychoanalysis, with its renewed emphasis on the needs of the community, would engage a broader swath of citizenry with simpler tools. We want a reduction in vengeance, not a therapeutic interlude that exalts the analyst.

Moss is persistent. He establishes a link to Fyodor Dostoevsky's (2002) famous *The Brothers Karamazov* and its account of Christ's encounter with the Grand Inquisitor. That interaction partially mimics the biblical description of the temptations of Jesus Christ found in the Gospels of Matthew, Mark, and Luke. Moss conjures up the turning of stone into bread, the question of Christ's protection by angels as he hurls himself from a height, and the offer of wealth in exchange for devil worship. After a long night of unsuccessful importuning by the Inquisitor, Jesus simply stands up, kisses the Inquisitor, and walks off. Moss (2017, p. 165) asks us: "What do we do about this kiss?" He agrees we could interpret it as a kind of forgiveness, a convenient package all neatly tied up by Christianity. If we know that the "kiss means forgiveness, we will also know what forgiveness means" (Moss 2017, p. 165).

Moss is toying with us. He points out that there is nothing certain about the kiss. After all, there is no commentary and no hints about its qualities or the intentions of the kisser. Nevertheless, in a strange twist, he notes that Christ strikes a posture of love and offers the possibility of a new beginning, one that sets us on the task of forgiving. Yes, Jesus appears to take a long time to reflect before walking away. However, I think the important point is to think more about the possibility of reflexive and impulsive charity, which mobilizes forgiveness.

# Francesc Tosquelles and the Art of Institutional Psychotherapy[9]

In the small, almost hidden American Folk Art Museum located on the Upper West Side of Manhattan, I recently attended a special exhibition focused on "Francesc (François) Tosquelles: Avant-Garde Psychiatry and the Birth of Art Brut." After the museum visit, I pursued other reading to sharpen his image and to understand better the context in which he had operated. His name has certainly attracted interest in the last decade or so. In an article in *Current Events*, the University of Barcelona's Joana Masó (2021) called Tosquelles a "transverse heterodox," where many pathways meet. She noted some of those paths: medicine, psychoanalysis, theater, poetry, cinema, and politics.

Francesc Tosquelles was born on August 22, 1912, in the Catalonia region of Spain. He studied medicine and psychiatry at the University of Barcelona and trained in psychoanalysis. During the Spanish Civil War (1936–1939), he served as psychiatric head of the Republican army. He was among thousands of civilians and military who sought refuge in the South of France during 1939. Wishing to deal harshly with these unwelcome socialists and anarchists, French authorities set up a labor-camp system for them. Tosquelles spent several months at the Septfonds camp, where he built a psychiatry unit based on therapeutic principles that he had developed while treating combatants on the front lines of the Spanish Civil War.

In early 1940, he was recruited to work at the psychiatric hospital in nearby Saint-Alban-sur-Limagnole, an isolated facility in the French department of Lozère. He worked there until 1962, developing a psychiatric practice that earned him praise, especially in France and Spain, regarding institutional psychiatry and its connection to art.

The American Folk Art Museum exhibition's curators suggested that Tosquelles was influenced by his experiences in the Spanish conflict, his time at Septfonds, and living in France during World War II. They maintained that, in Tosquelles's view, war conditions had a significant effect on patients and the hospital itself. The collaborationist French Vichy government participated in the labeling of psychiatric populations as undesirable, which helped bring about some of

---

[9] Adapted with permission from Griffith EEH: Francesc Tosquelles and the Art of Institutional Psychotherapy. *Psychiatric News*, October 2024. Copyright © 2024 American Psychiatric Association. All rights reserved.

Tosquelles's creative changes and also led to the use of Saint-Alban in support of members of the French Resistance and individuals hiding from the Nazis.

Tosquelles experimented with interventions intended to impact medicotherapeutic, political, and sociocultural spheres. In today's terms, he saw the needs of individual patients while also grasping the necessity of making changes at the organizational-practice level of the hospital. This meant changes in attitudes and postures of hospital personnel and administrators. It was no accident, then, that the presence of the conflict in Spain, which connected itself so effortlessly to events elsewhere in Europe and concretely in France, would have had such an effect on Tosquelles. War, and specifically fascism, was a root cause of human suffering and displacement, produced alienation of human beings from one another and from their social environment, and caused different forms of psychopathology.

Examples of new changes that came to Saint-Alban were training of caretakers and nuns in basic psychiatry; establishment of nonhierarchical relations among patients, medical staff, and neighbors from the village; and encouragement of patients' creativity. Other changes included freer movement between town and hospital, produced by destruction of the hospital's walls, and permission for patients to engage in paid employment in the village. Thus, as Annika Olsen (2024) noted in her critique of the exhibition on the Artnet website, patients were included in daily activities such as maintaining the hospital. They also had access to a library, cinema, and art workshops, in addition to use of a space where different types of celebrations, plays, and dances were held. These composite changes became known as institutional psychotherapy.

Writing about the exhibition in *The New York Times*, Travis Diehl (2024) reminded us that the art collector Jean Dubuffet visited Saint-Alban in 1945 seeking examples of the art produced by the hospital's patients. Dubuffet had previously seen some of the works in Paris and was interested in building a collection of this "art brut"—the work of patients who had not been contaminated by formal art training. Saint-Alban had conserved the work of several of its resident artists, such as Auguste Forestier (Figure 3.5) and Marguerite Sirvins (Figure 3.6). Dubuffet was committed to stripping this art of its earlier stigmatizing label promoted by some psychiatric hospitals: "psychopathological art." That label suggested a linkage between artistic styles and certain psychiatric conditions.

*Facing Disability*

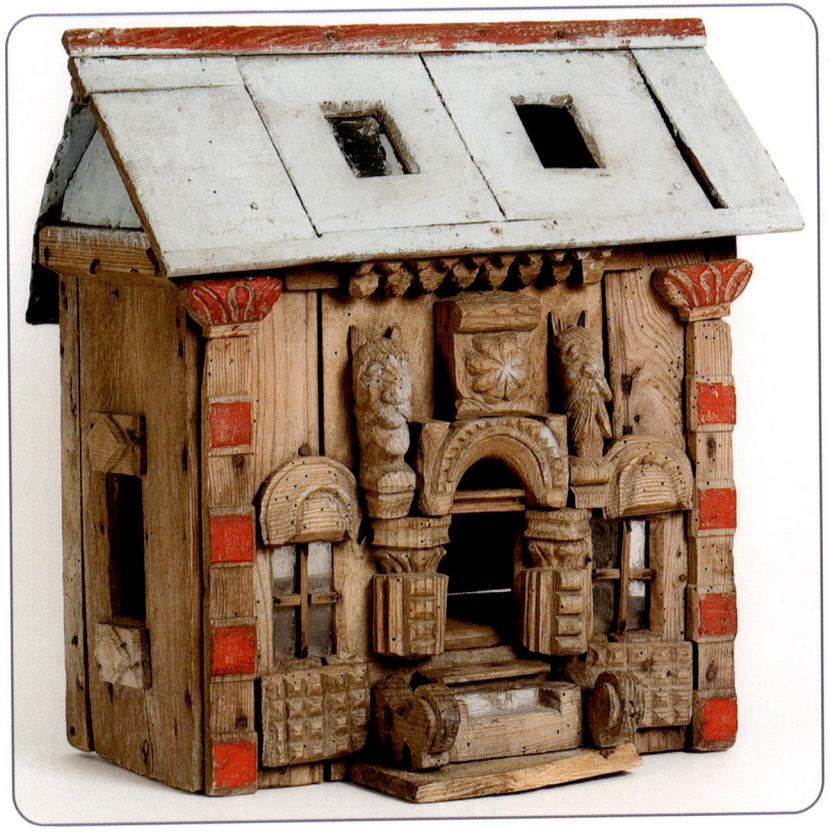

**Figure 3.5** Untitled (House With Two Carved Heads) n.d., by Auguste Forestier (1887–1958, France).

Sculpture: Wood, metal, glass, paint, colored pencil. 43 x 45 x 31.5 cm. No inv. 2009.3.1.

*Source.* LaM/Lille métropole musée d'art moderne, d'art contemporain et d'art brut, Villeneuve d'Ascq, France. Copyright photographique: Cécile Dubart.

Not surprisingly, Tosquelles was more interested in patients' art as a path to rehabilitation and readaptation to a social reality that facilitated healing. The debate also continued concerning the ownership and meaning of this form of work product that took on economic value through individuals like Dubuffet. I can barely imagine the debates provoked by Tosquelles, a psychoanalyst and intellectual who interacted with many visitors to Saint-Alban, such as the Surrealist poet Paul Éluard and the French psychoanalyst Frantz Fanon. Those discussions

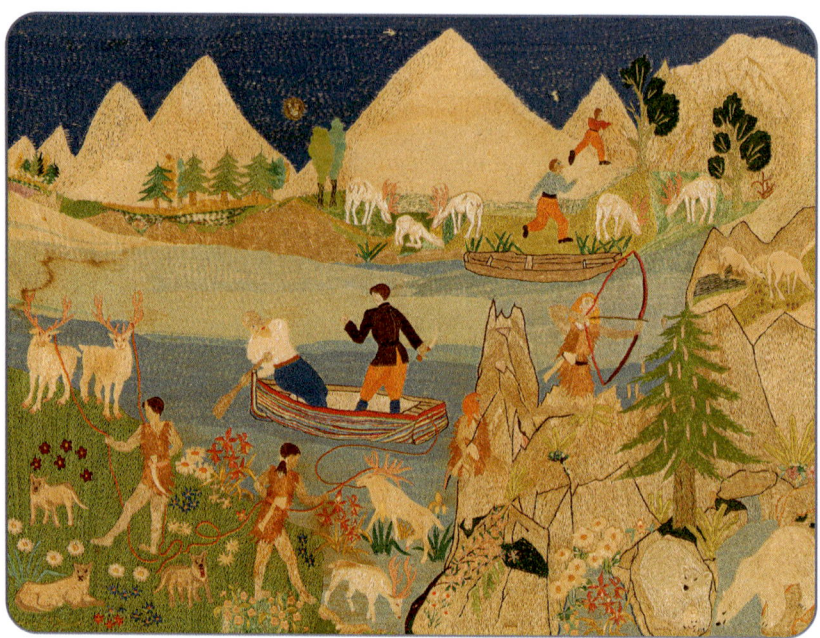

**Figure 3.6** Landscape With Boats, Hunters, and Animals c. 1944–1955 by Marguerite Sirvins (1890–1957, France).

Oeuvre textile: Rayon thread embroidered on fabric. 60 x 80 x 2 cm. No inv. 2018.10.4.

*Source.* LaM/Lille métropole musée d'art moderne, d'art contemporain et d'art brut, Villeneuve d'Ascq, France. Copyright photographique: Nicolas Dewitte/LaM.

must have been something to behold. The integration of village, hospital, literary and art movements, psychoanalysis, and war was never part of my lived experience.

*Facing Disability*

# Comments and Clinical Observations

An intriguing aspect of this text is that columns were often written in isolation from one another, reflecting principally what was taking place in the broader society, at home and overseas. Yet, groups of them could naturally be brought together to represent separate themes within the context of people, places, and health. In this chapter, from different angles I frame a discussion of how disease and health disorders affect our capacities to contend with daily life. The experience of being sick often leaves us with some sort of disability, a particular difficulty carrying out certain tasks. There is the inability to see or hear, the lack of control over emotions, the problem of managing our behavior, the inability to walk or climb stairs, and so on. The list is extensive, ranging from less or more serious, to ephemeral or permanent, to responsive or not responsive to treatment. In every instance, one of the therapeutic tasks is to try hard to help the patient return to participating in activities of daily living and to enjoying the privileges of citizenship.

This chapter's first column discusses a public exhibition about deafness that I attended during a 2019 trip to Paris. The advertisement of the retrospective made me realize instantly how little I knew about the Deaf community of any country. Recognizing this, I included a session on Deaf persons when I first developed a course in cultural psychiatry at Yale. For that meeting with the residents, I invited a colleague who had a Deaf child. She was willing to discuss her experience raising her family while learning about the culture of the Deaf community. She helped the trainees and me cultivate a curiosity about the phenomenon of being hearing impaired. I have not met many psychiatrists who are familiar with the daily lives of people in this community, their struggles with identity development, and their efforts to fit into the hearing world.

I began the column by describing my experience playing soccer with a teammate who could neither speak nor hear. The other players welcomed him warmly, and he was pleased that he had overcome his disability and could play the game at our level. An occasional problem cropped up when he committed a foul, and the referee whistled to stop play. Unable to hear, he continued running with the ball. Another member of our team then had to explain to the referee why our teammate had not obeyed the signal. The referee always quickly calmed down, impressed that our friend with his hearing disability could compete effectively against other players who could hear all that was taking place on the field. I never had the chance to ask my teammate about his life history. However, it was apparent that he had not given up his boyhood dream of being a competitive player well into adulthood.

I was also proud of my teammates. They did not stigmatize him on the field. When I gave him the pass from which he scored, he was in the position to receive the ball. Once in that location, I was obligated to send the ball through to him. Making the pass was recognizing what he had done. That is what everyone with a disability asks of neighbors. After the game, he came to me smiling radiantly and just bowed, silently acknowledging that I had assisted with his goal. It was well after that match, in reflecting on disability and the world of the Deaf community, that I concluded that he wanted his teammates to see past the disability and welcome him as a talented adult player. Like all of us, he wanted to belong to the group and to be defined by his playing, not by his disability. This is an important reminder to clinicians of the mindset required of them as they approach their patients.

In the second column, I discussed Professor Larry Davidson's (2018) work and his contributions to the concept of recovery in mental health. Davidson relied on an earlier definition of *recovery*, provided by Patricia Deegan (1988), which alluded to the real-life experience of those who accept and try to overcome the problems linked to mental illness. These individuals also find themselves experiencing a renewed sense of personal identity. They work to overcome or adapt to the limitations imposed by the disability. In my example of the soccer player, as well as in my description of the visitors at the French exhibition on Deaf persons, I observed people who refused to let their disability tie them down in a way that classed them as victims. Still, Davidson (2003) made clear in his text on living outside mental illness that many factors may affect the outcome of those struggling with psychiatric disorders. Ultimately, Davidson (2003, p. 50) argued that the risk was "too great not to believe in the potential of every person for recovery," to some degree, from psychiatric disorders. This helps with the task of providing hope to the patient.

Davidson and his Yale team contributed over several years to improving public/community psychiatry. In the mid-1970s, I was in psychiatric training at New York City's Lincoln Hospital, as I described in the 5th column of this chapter, "Memories of a Community Hospital." That was the era of community psychiatry, and I observed, from that vantage point, shifts in the structure of mental health services. Local programs and communities received federal money for psychiatric service delivery. In that fashion, Lincoln Hospital delivered acute short-term inpatient services and emergency services, while the Lincoln Community Mental Health Center directed a day hospital and outpatient services in several community clinics. This period de-emphasized state-hospital services and accentuated a broad spectrum of services delivered in the community. In addition, as I pointed out, there was an explicit assurance that community representatives would have a voice in the organization of the services. Davidson (2003) emphasized the role of what he called a consumer movement in service organization. I suspect that the mixture of community advocates and consumers/survivors varied depending on the community. At Lincoln, the physicians were provided by contract through a local medical school. The ensuing complexities that flowed from this administrative reality are well described by Gabriel Koz (2021), as I stated in the column about Lincoln Hospital.

I make these points about the community mental health center (CMHC) movement to emphasize that deinstitutionalization had started by the early 1970s in programs where I worked. And notions of rehabilitation had begun to reappear in discussions of what one wanted for the patient contending with mental illness. I emphasize "reappear" because the last column in this chapter points out that Francesc Tosquelles had by 1940 been thinking about the recovery of psychiatric patients, their autonomous privileges in the hospital, and their reintegration into local communities.

Davidson (2003) emphasized that ideas about the chronicity and downward evolution of psychotic disorders, what he called the Kraepelinian view of schizophrenia, were responsible for the pessimistic conclusion regarding the eventual outcome of these disorders. Although this negative view, coming from the academic world, had its effect on psychiatric practice, I have always believed that other factors in the social arena had their own influences on perceptions of psychiatric patients. Theorizing about the developmental trends in psychiatry has often ignored its linkage to other historic dimensions of the external social world. When the federal government offered money to undergird psychiatric and substance abuse services, medical schools were not enthusiastic about entering this arena of activity. Furthermore, the requirement that community services be established with community input was never excitedly accepted and welcomed by medical schools. This was a readily observable aspect of university/community relations in my experience. And these interactions generally worsened when the relationships were racialized. The connection of outcome to notions of dignity-enhancing care was not an inherent element in the foundation of community services.

It was a remarkable event in my initial professional life that I went from the Lincoln Hospital/Community Mental Health Center psychiatry training program to an academic post at Yale School of Medicine. It is in the latter context that Professor Davidson espoused his notions of recovery and tried his best to apply his ideas both nationally and internationally. At Yale, with his eye on a positive outcome for psychiatric disorders, he emphasized the importance of integrating community living into a structured treatment plan whenever possible. This was different from accenting institutional options as a first preference without first imagining the possibility of the psychiatric patient's future as a citizen of some community. Reintegration into community life was more likely to ensure that the individual would enjoy the privileges experienced by the average citizen. Spending one's life in an institution undermined the promises of citizenship and made it difficult to see the benefits of rehabilitation.

It may appear that what I have just described was straightforwardly simple to implement. It was not. Many academics resented nonmedical professionals' participation in the formulation of treatment plans. The idea that the patient was at the center of treatment planning and should therefore provide structured input was hard for the established biomedical system. There was also another fly in the ointment. Someone started circulating the myth that outpatient care would be much cheaper than hospital care. This idea was snapped up by legislators and led to unexpected problems. Many of the seriously ill patients needed to be housed, supervised in their activities of daily living, and offered exercises that would sharpen their skills in different domains and develop them in others. In this context, caregiving in the community became an expensive process, especially because it was quickly recognized that no two patients had the same needs. Then, confusion over the meaning of recovery provided its own unmanageable mess. Administrators thought that everybody would simply become cured in these outpatient clinics, obtain work, and rent nice apartments.

Recovery theorists, on the other hand, were talking about principles like "redefining self and accepting illness ...overcoming stigma, renewing a sense of hope and commitment, ... managing one's symptoms, being supported by others, being involved in meaningful activities and expanded social roles" (Davidson 2003, p. 45). This meant that psychiatric care required new familiarity with matters of housing, rehabilitation, vocational training, public transportation, public health maintenance, and substance use. This chapter includes two columns about an outpatient clinic's rehabilitation activities in the domain of writing. That clinic also offered activities in painting and music. Publishing the patients' writing in *The Beacon*, a formal publication, made both patients and staff feel proud of the final product. I mentioned the focus on promoting trust and fostering community in the writing groups. It is intriguing, too, how individuals can use their imagination in the task of writing and formulating ideas. Patients have the additional opportunity to sharpen identity and get beyond the sense of being disabled in broad spheres of living as opposed to struggling with more narrow areas of disability. In a separate column, focused on patients' art that is curated within the museum of Sainte-Anne Hospital in Paris, I discussed the potential promise that patients' creative activities can offer when pushed to a high level of accomplishment that is supported by the facility.

With regard to end-of-year rituals and making promises for the future, I wondered how patients with significant disability from mental illness take part in such events. Perhaps the first test is to focus one's mind on the positive things that have happened during the past year. Then one can try to develop a sense of gratitude and proceed to figure out what factors or elements can be mobilized to start the new year with confidence—that one has a chance of repeating positive things in the coming year. We all know that when the old year has not been good, one can become preoccupied with the negative side of things as the clock slides into the new year.

This is why I consider the column on forgiveness so relevant here. It reminded me, as I wrote it, of the patients who asked me, especially when they were in the throes of acute exacerbations of their illness, whether God was angry with them. They wanted to know how to pursue forgiveness. They sought communion with someone or some force that could sustain them as they entered that new year, uncertain but needy and dependent. They hoped that the passage from the old to the new could signal some sense of transformation, a relinquishing of the worst symptoms, and arrival of the evidence of incipient recovery. Disability has become a stigmatizing marker of psychiatric illness that contributes to creating a context in which oppression takes place. While one individual experiences oppression along the axis of gender, another patient contends with it on the axis of race. Yet another feels it in the context of disabling mental illness that eats at patients' autonomy and feeds the sense of privilege and superiority of clinicians who have the power in the biomedical system. I suggest here that treating professionals should avoid this potential pitfall.

Some years ago, when I was invited to take up the post of medical director in Connecticut's Department of Mental Health and Addiction Services, I decided to focus on improving both the quality of services and the linkages among service centers. It took at least a year to popularize the notion that both arms of the mission were equally important. In some centers, while clinicians worked hard on the quality of the work they saw as strictly psychiatric, they attended less to the needs of the patient in the arenas of housing, vocational services, or dental care. I am not arguing here that clinicians must personally attend to these tasks. However, I am recommending that they recognize the importance of this work that benefits the patient. Clinicians can add their support to ensure that other colleagues trained in these arenas become members of the treatment team.

I appreciated that a mental health professional, trained and prepared to provide some form of verbal therapy, may not rush to delve into these other areas. However, an eye must remain on the patient's capacity to deal with the tasks of everyday living. This observation was especially important in the case of those individuals who were seriously and chronically ill. As a result, clinicians had to think more broadly and holistically about the psychiatric patient served in the public sector. As the patient entered the service door of inpatient or outpatient services, the question was: What did the patient need? This focus demanded some understanding of the individual's functioning. The next step was to determine the required services and their location. Every service center did not provide a complete range of services. That reality forced us to think seriously about the interconnectedness of services or what others prefer to call the coordination of services. Administrative and clinical service coordination became an important part of the work, required expanded budgets, and squarely accentuated the meaning of rehabilitation and recovery. This wave of change also catalyzed revised curricula for training mental health professionals.

Let us take, for example, the capacity to handle one's money each day. Those working in clinical psychiatry must appreciate that numerous skills are required for success in independent living. Those skills may be affected negatively by psychiatric disorders of all sorts. In addition, hospital stays often lead to atrophy or loss of some capacities. Traumatic experiences, especially those that lead to reduced everyday activity or prolonged dysfunction, can also alter one's ability to perform certain acts. That is why I emphasized the notion of rehabilitation in this chapter. Some clinicians forget to spend time inquiring about their patients' activities and falsely conclude that once patients keep clinic appointments, they are fulfilling adequately their roles as community citizens. Curiosity about how patients spend their days reveals from time to time that isolation is a significant part of their lives.

Reducing patients' isolation is important because it aids movement of the mind and body. Nevertheless, it must be balanced against the imperative of respect for patients' wishes. Clinicians have the potential to disrespect patients because they expect patients to recognize that clinicians are recommending what is good for them. I remember the case of one patient who repeatedly preferred his independence and isolation to what he considered as intrusive home visits from his case manager. Resolving this matter required extensive discussion, because the patient was clearly able to present his wishes quietly and logically. Another patient, before being discharged from inpatient care, declared thoughtfully that he would return to his lifestyle of visiting a certain female friend with whom he used drugs. This patient's family always stayed in contact with him and consistently attended his discharge planning meetings. They insisted that he be kept in the hospital involuntarily or be considered for involuntary outpatient commitment.

Griffith and Papapietro (2018) have discussed the complexity of such cases and the need to have an established way of ensuring thoughtful debate. I point out that in the second situation, the patient's attorney and family members were present at planning meetings. The discussion included consideration of different treatment options. This clinical review should not be confused with a formal legal hearing presided over by a probate judge. In some jurisdictions, the patient's attorney may attend clinical team meetings. This is a unique feature of public psychiatry in some areas. In my view, it adds substantially to the dignity of the review process and opens the review so that the patient's wishes receive serious consideration. In this instance, the patient's preferences did not coincide with those of his family. The result was an eye-opening debate about the meaning of autonomy and decision-making. In this situation, the patient was judged to be handling the conversation as effectively as everyone else in the room.

## Questions to Ponder

1. Do you agree with the notion that people with psychiatric disabilities should first be given the opportunity to live in the community?
2. Do you prefer that an individual's disability be made visible to others or that it be hidden if possible?
3. Should consumers of care be invited to offer input into the design of clinical service systems?
4. Is it helpful to contemplate past experiences before planning for the next year?
5. Do you think forgiveness would be useful in solving differences between governments?

## References

Cohen J: Facing Fear [documentary short film]. Jason Cohen Productions, 2014

Davidson L: Is there a future for recovery? World Association for Psychosocial Rehabilitation Bulletin, December 2018. Available at: https://www.wapr.org/bulletin-archive/released-wapr-bulletin-no-42. Accessed July 8, 2024.

Davidson L: Living Outside Mental Illness: Qualitative Stories of Recovery in Schizophrenia. New York, New York University Press, 2003

Deegan P: Recovery: the lived experience of rehabilitation. Psychosoc Rehabil J 11(4):11–19, 1988

Diehl T: The avant-garde psychiatrist who built an artistic refuge. New York Times, July 19, 2024

Dostoevsky F: The Brothers Karamazov, 12th Edition. Translated by Pevear R, Volokhonsky L. New York, Farrar, Straus & Giroux, 2002

Griffith EEH: Visibility in a psychiatric hospital's museum. Psychiatric News, December 31, 2019

Griffith EEH: Creative writing and psychiatric rehabilitation. Psychiatric News, April 1, 2021

Griffith EEH, Papapietro D: Forensic ethics and involuntary outpatient commitment, in Ethics Challenges in Forensic Psychiatry and Psychology Practice. Edited by Griffith EEH. New York, Columbia University Press, 2018, pp 116–131

Hart A: From multicultural competence to radical openness: a psychoanalytic engagement of otherness. American Psychoanalyst 51(1):12–27, 2017

Kaplan SR, Roman M: The Organization and Delivery of Mental Health Services in the Ghetto: The Lincoln Hospital Experience. New York, Praeger, 1973

Koz G: Made in South Africa: A Psychiatrist's Journey. Petersburg, VA, Dietz Press, 2021

Masó J: Tosquelles, the forgotten subversive psychiatrist. Current Events, May 27, 2021

Moss D: After the offense: thoughts on forgiveness, in At War With the Obvious: Disruptive Thinking in Psychoanalysis. New York, Routledge, 2017, pp 153–167

Olsen A: Inside the 20th-century French psychiatric hospital that saw the birth of art brut. Artnet, July 23, 2024

Ozarin LD: Review of The Organization and Delivery of Mental Health Services in the Ghetto: The Lincoln Hospital Experience—by Seymour R. Kaplan, M.D., and Melvin Roman, Ph.D.; Praeger, New York City, 1973, 315 pages, $19.50. Psychiatr Serv 25(7):477–479, 1974

Philips D, Linington L, Penman D: Writing Well: Creative Writing and Mental Health. Philadelphia, PA, Jessica Kingsley, 1999

Thomas CS: Review of The Organization and Delivery of Mental Health Services. Am J Public Health 64(8):821, 1974

# 4

# Confronting the COVID-19 Pandemic

# Columns From *Psychiatric News*

## Building Community: We Gatherin' Barbados[1]

It was a beautiful February morning in 2020. I had never witnessed a church ceremony like this one, whose objective was the solemnization of citizens' coming together and celebrating their national cohesion. The Barbados government called it a "gatherin'," dropping the last letter of the word to signify that the term was formulated in the people's street patois. The government began this unique yearlong initiative a month earlier in St. Lucy, the most northern parish of this Caribbean country. A St. Lucy contingent was now passing the baton to the people in the neighboring parish of St. Peter. The country's governor general was in attendance, as were the acting prime minister, several parliamentary representatives, and individuals from all walks of Barbadian life. Tropical flora decorated the Anglican church, and the music was decidedly ecumenical. People wore outfits reflecting the melding of their British, African, and West Indian cultural heritage, as illustrated by the women's headwear in Figure 4.1. There has been, of course, dynamic cultural change in their customs and rituals since Barbados obtained independence from its centuries-old British colonizers in 1966.

The government invited all Bajans, the diminutive name for Barbadians, to celebrate themselves throughout 2020. All 11 parishes of Barbados will, in turn, welcome residents from other parishes. Bajans throughout the diaspora have also been invited home to celebrate the island, its culture, and its people's achievements. The objective, given the symbolism of the year 2020, is to gather and simultaneously look back and forward.

The organizers of the gatherin' have been advertising a range of activities. For example, sports will be represented by dominoes and road tennis. Public lectures will focus on different aspects of the island's socioeconomic and infrastructural development. There will

---

[1] This column was composed in early 2020 and highlighted the spirit of hope and positivity that preceded the arrival of the pandemic.

Adapted with permission from Griffith EEH: Building Community: We Gatherin' Barbados. *Psychiatric News*, April 2020. Copyright © 2020 American Psychiatric Association. All rights reserved.

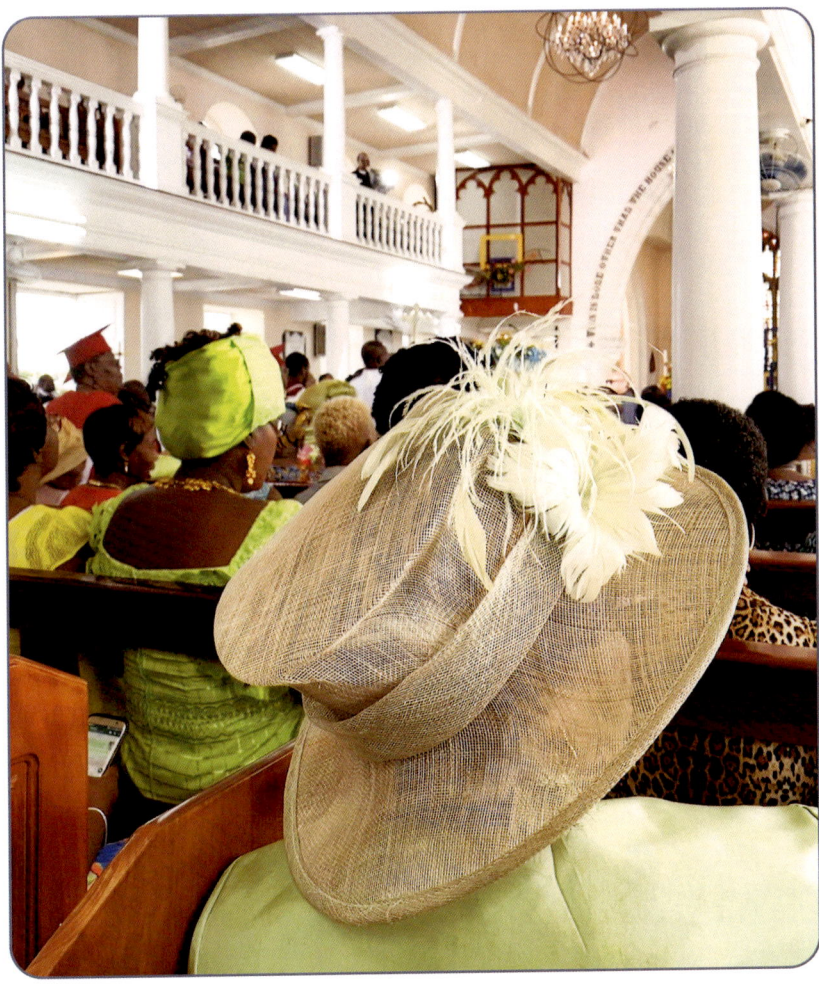

**Figure 4.1** Congregants Wearing Hats at a Public Service, St. Peter Parish Church, Barbados.

The photograph illustrates the melding of their British, African, and West Indian cultural heritage.

*Source.* Photograph by Brigitte Griffith.

also be tours of the island's patrimony and discussions of the country's artists, economists, and health caregivers. Steel pan music and calypso singing will be juxtaposed against the island's heritage and traditions of classical and church music. Even genealogists will be available to help in finding one's roots.

There was little doubt the gatherin' was meant to be inclusive. That's why the activity venues extended into all the parishes, and the themes of the individual meetings covered the old, the young, males and females, and broad interests of the population. One could tell that there was a sense of healing in the air. Everybody was promoting interpersonal connection, pride in self and country, awareness of what it means to be a Barbadian, and confidence in self and neighbors. The politicians devised this ingenious way of inviting everybody to renew membership in the small country and contemplate ways of sharpening the connection to home. Added to that invitation was the prod to take some responsibility for the future of the island and its efforts to confront the growing drug problem, violence, and unemployment.

In the weeks following the Sunday service, I chatted with local and returning folk. I visited the countryside and sampled food in restaurants. I attended steel pan concerts and toured art museums. I even revisited museums and listened to the crashing of the waves at different beaches. I remembered Devika Chawla's (2015) advice to monitor and untangle home's habits and its affective rhythms. There was also Chawla's mention of the personal restorative power of home's rituals and performances. I could see home in music, art, sports, religious ritual, and the smells and sights of Bajan life all around me.

There must be something good about celebrating oneself, one's roots, and the contributions of family to a firm developmental foundation. I liked the notion that home space could symbolize achievement and promise. This was a Barbadian form of civic engagement and community building, with significant implications for individual and collective well-being.

## My Fable of Contagion[2]

Jill Lepore (2020) started her narrative about the devastating effects of plague and other epidemics with a harsh reminder: "Stories of epidemics are stories of language made powerless and man made brute." My fable of contagion is no different, although it starts with me, sitting peacefully in a Barbados Anglican church in early March, enjoying a Sunday morning service. The sunlight streamed through the large windows, and I could hear roosters crowing in the country

---

[2] Adapted with permission from Griffith EEH: My Fable of Contagion. *Psychiatric News*, May 2020. Copyright © 2020 American Psychiatric Association. All rights reserved.

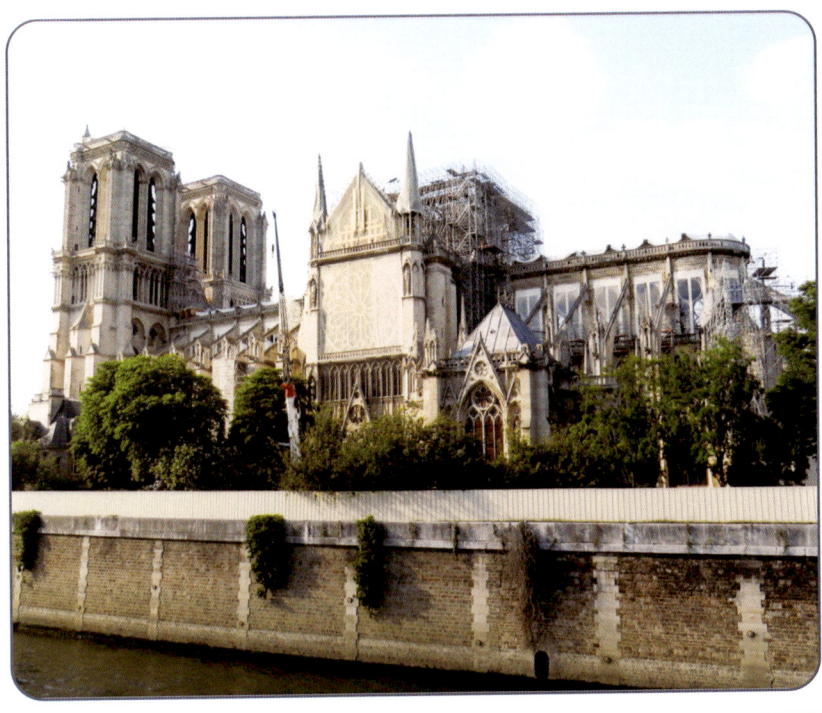

**Figure 4.2** Notre Dame Cathedral, Paris, France.

The photograph shows the severe damage caused by the April 2019 fire.

*Source.* Photograph by R. C. Grantham, AIA.

churchyard. I realized that the rector was explaining two new diocesan decisions related to COVID-19. In administering the Holy Eucharist, priests would distribute only the bread, and there would be no wine to celebrate the gift of His blood. The communal chalice was forbidden. Additionally, the handshakes and hugs that occurred after the priest intoned "May the peace of the Lord be with you" would be no longer permitted. COVID-19 had struck, with little fuss perhaps, but with immeasurable impact. Some days later, the authorities closed sacred spaces, part of the strategy of keeping us apart and blunting the nefarious effects of this virus.

I perceived this transformation of the sacred space as violent, even though I understood the public health rationale of interrupting contagion. It reminded me of my feelings a year ago when fire destroyed a part of the Notre Dame Cathedral in Paris (Figure 4.2), leaving the building looking lifeless and abandoned. When sacred spaces that highlight the inherent beauty and peace around us are suddenly absent, it feels destructive and pointless. The absence means no preaching, singing, resting, meditating, reading of the Word, or even complaining; my sense of community was shocked.

I read a striking report by Raphaëlle Bacqué and Ariane Chemin (2020) that described the outcome of a religious Lenten retreat organized by the Open Door Christian Church, an evangelical Protestant movement. About 2,000 individuals attended the meeting in Mulhouse, France, between February 17 and 24, 2020. By the last day, several attendees started complaining of flulike symptoms, and they tested positive for the coronavirus. Many were hospitalized, and several died.

In another account from *Le Monde*, Gérard Méjean and Solenn de Royer (2020) talked of a group of 11 Capuchin monks still operating in a French monastery. After a predatory visit by this virus, six now remain. These examples of gratuitous attacks on sacred spaces fall, my friends tell me, into the category of theodicy. That is where the learned inquire about God's place in all this suffering, and we question God's silence and whether He has abandoned us or is mocking and punishing us. It is where we cry, "How long, O Lord, how long?"

Believers aren't just frightened by the onslaught of the pandemic. There is a surreal fear that comes from an inability to contend with God's silence as we seek dialogue. Pugnaciously questioning Him leaves me feeling guilty and helpless. Inevitably, I give up and conclude that my arms are too short to box with God. In this instance, too, science offers no simple solutions. Uncertainty is rampant. Respiratory distress syndrome is a theoretical conundrum. Statistical curves are being flattened and sharpened and interpreted differently by academic groups.

I like the question I heard framed by a preacher in an Easter Sunday service that was streaming from an empty New York City church. "What do we do with the suffering?" The answer came from a pastor friend who told me patiently that I need faith and should put God in control amid the confusion. The friend also pointed out that I should understand God's role in helping us medical professionals contend with COVID-19. While I ponder these deep matters of theodicy, I keep putting energy into improving the beneficent nature of the new spaces we are occupying. I can see the special beauty and simplicity in caring for neighbors. I hope this melding of the religious and the physician will get us through.

A Catholic psychiatrist told me of Teilhard de Chardin's prayer (de Chardin 2010) "Patient Trust": "Above all, trust in the slow work of God

..." and give Him the benefit of believing that He is leading us. It is a way of developing patience, trust, and acceptance of the uncertain journey we all must make.

## Expressions of Loss and Hope[3]

When I was a schoolboy, I had to recite a geographic truth constantly. It was that Barbados was shaped like a shoulder of mutton, with its narrow end marking the north of the island. The land at that very tip was called North Point (Figure 4.3). It was flat and dry and seemingly abandoned. Standing on that ground was like being on a cliff looking way out to sea. On a sunny day, the water was a deep blue maelstrom of interactive currents, contrasting sharply with the white, foamy waves crashing on the rocks below.

Whenever I return home, I make the pilgrimage to North Point. On the way there, in the last mile or so, I go past St. Swithin's Anglican Church, named after an Anglo-Saxon bishop from the 5th century. The name seems incongruous with an Antillean country village. Still, every time the church comes into view, I decide afresh that it marks the entrance to this utterly beautiful area, desolate in a certain way, even deathly quiet at times. The vista of the sea, the salty breeze competing with the imposing warmth from the sun, and the occasional sheep or goat roaming unimpeded and owning the territory create an improbable landscape. I love my connection to this place.

I have had to return to memories like this during the last few months, as the coronavirus has rambunctiously forced me to seek refuge from its rampage. Several friends have told me of their personal experiences with confinement to home. The boundaries of the space seem to close in, making the square footage progressively smaller and turning home into what Professor Chester Pierce used to call an extreme environment. The perceived change limits movement and imposes a new monotony that can be frightening. My friends complain of being cut off from familiar support networks and landscapes. They dislike the isolation and miss the consistency and reliability offered by their pre-pandemic lifestyles. They describe a feeling of stark isolation and an inability to master their small spaces and their energy and mobility. One might say they no longer feel at home in their restructured

---

[3] Adapted with permission from Griffith EEH: Expressions of Loss and Hope. *Psychiatric News*, June 2020. Copyright © 2020 American Psychiatric Association. All rights reserved.

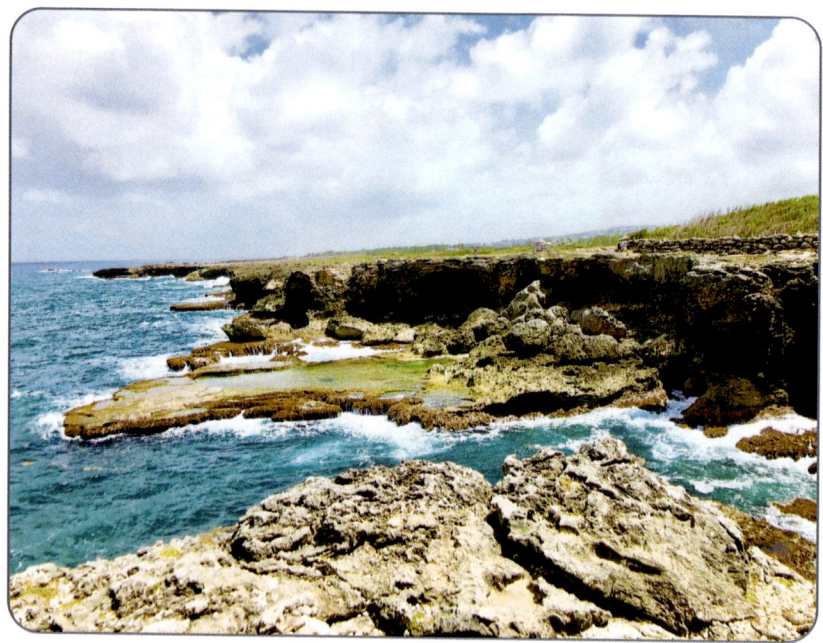

**Figure 4.3** North Point, Barbados.

This area lies at the most northern tip of the island.

*Source.* Photograph by Brigitte Griffith.

homes. They have been exiled from outside to the inside. Homes can be cocoons of comfort. The pandemic mocks that claim.

Pierce emphasized two other elements in conceptualizing the extreme environment. The first is amorphous structure. This refers to our need for some orderliness and predictability in our average day, as well as our frustration caused by the contradictory advice about the virus that bombards us daily. The second element, indefinite stays, frames the uncertainty about when the confinement will end, which worsens our anxiety. A feeling of abandonment sometimes takes over, and we become hypervigilant. As I contemplated all this while reminiscing about my dialogues with Chester Pierce described in *Race and Excellence* (Griffith 2023), it struck me that the accounts of present concerns linked to the coronavirus sound like tales of exile. Most prominent is the loss of pleasant remembrances focused on planning for the future.

I try to hold on to my memories of North Point, where I always feel so relaxed and untethered, waiting for ancestral voices to whisper in my ear and grateful for the chance to savor nature's elegance. I conclude that there are some magnificent places on earth, even on a little island in the Caribbean. At North Point, incidentally, there is now a small restaurant overlooking the water. I enjoy its blackbelly sheep stew with rice and the bread pudding for dessert. Souvenirs of pilgrimages to these distinctive places of safety and freedom can be an antidote to extreme environments.

Frauke Josenhans (2017), the editor of *Artists in Exile: Expressions of Loss and Hope*, discussed the problem of being separated from what is familiar to us. While we become preoccupied in the new space with the imagery of loss and alienation, restorative nostalgia can help us reimagine home and reinvigorate our resilience.

## Contemplating Changes From a Transformative Year[4]

I spent the first two and a half months of 2020 in Barbados. That is where, for those accustomed to it, the sun warms from the inside out. The night air is reassuringly cooled by the sea. Derek Walcott (2004), the Caribbean poet, noted that in such places, a fierce thirst can transform iced water into a gasping benediction. It was easy to strike a pose of contentment in my island home, with the daily rhythms of life so easy and relaxed. I was in good health and in possession of enough resources to be confident that the next meal was assured. I was jogging several miles most afternoons at a public track located on the coast near the beach. Sunsets were full of vibrant colors occasionally punctuated by a rainbow. Not all the day's hours were idle. I was home, and I could take delight in a mere drizzle. I had time to contemplate the blackbirds every morning trying to steal some crumbs fallen from my slice of coconut bread.

In mid-March 2020, things changed. I returned to New Haven, Connecticut, and life "up North," as they say in the islands. A few days later, I confronted the lockdown. If Barbados had been fueling my feelings of immortality, the pandemic reawakened concerns of vulnerability. I remember the increasing attention to what I could do within the confines of a comfortable apartment: read, listen to music,

---

[4] Adapted with permission from Griffith EEH: Contemplating Changes From a Transformative Year. *Psychiatric News*, February 2021. Copyright © 2021 American Psychiatric Association. All rights reserved.

write, make music with my steel pan, watch television, talk to family members, and think. Reading daily newspapers brought into sharp relief the fierceness of COVID-19. Accounts of the deaths among the religious in French monasteries were frightening. There was a special coldness about the pileup of coffins in New York and Italian cities that left bystanders gasping for air.

Claire Marin, a French philosopher, has had some recent thoughts about the changes caused by the pandemic. These were reported by Nicolas Truong (2020) from an interview with the philosopher. Marin suggested that the sacrifices imposed by hardship and suffering at the hands of the pandemic might be attenuated by the benefits and improvements found in the new postpandemic reality. However, she recognized that there may not be a clear separation between the periods before and after the pandemic. Perhaps we may slip gradually into a new style of life, with calm periods and the occasional crisis. Marin theorized that we may simply have to prepare ourselves to live differently.

She did have specific concerns related to technological progress. We have all noticed the newly ubiquitous presence of videoconferencing, with its loss of eye contact and a sense of closeness. Gone may be the related recognizing of the other. She lamented the resulting impoverishment of human relationships, the diminished fluidity and spontaneity of human contact. She agreed that some of us may experience this sort of technological arrangement as a kind of liberation and may claim that it increases work productivity. We may even boast that it facilitates multitasking. However, she warned of the potential conflating of private and professional spaces, intimate and social exchanges. Ultimately, our private lives will suffer.

Marin questioned the diminution of "presence" in these virtual interactions. She saw presence as a dynamic element, as attention and momentum toward the other. We know it as a factor in the relationship between doctor and patient. She pointed out that technological advances reduce geographic distances. They also may increase psychological distance. Another important consideration is that technological advancement in communication has put patients' complaints too much in the public sphere, sometimes making the experience of illness humiliating and degrading. Marin recommended that we take note of the changes, for better and for worse. Then, we must move cautiously in determining what we will keep, especially among those changes that affect working, caregiving, and the ways in which we relate to others. Of course, other observers have made observations about the pandemics' effects. Geoff Dyer (2020) did so from the position of an Englishman living in America.

## Angels and the Pandemic[5]

It has been more than a year since we began living with the COVID-19 pandemic. I assume we marked the anniversary in different ways: through our individualized associations, ruminations about what we missed and what has changed, and thoughts about the transformations in our lives. Some of us may have knelt at a real or virtual altar, satisfied at having made it through and looking cautiously to a future. Others may have complained, because of the pain or from habit. I noticed a tenacious anger at times, in retaliation against COVID's insistence that it had an unmerciful mind of its own. From the beginning, the virus made clear that we were not in charge of this rampaging event.

The year was at times oppressive, brutal, even punitive. Despite the turmoil around them, some people maintained an equanimity of spirit. They offered comforting words, made conciliatory gestures, and radiated peace. I admired and celebrated the two women I know who telephoned each other regularly and engaged in mutual prayerful support. There was, too, my younger colleague who invited me to take walks with him on occasion. We discussed all sorts of subjects, enjoyed the human contact, and contemplated how best to continue trying to make this world better.

Thinking about these special individuals led me to private reveries about similar people and places. On one such excursion, I was back in the Army. It was a long time ago, in the early 1960s. I was engaged in research on bubonic plague at the Pasteur Institute in Saigon. It was my job to determine the kind of rat that carried the fleas capable of transmitting the disease to humans.

On the institute's campus, there was a small pavilion that served as a clinic for individuals with another historic ailment, sometimes called the plague of leprosy. In the Old Testament book of Leviticus at Chapter 14, one can find detailed descriptions of the rituals used to deal with this disease and its social implications. I have some familiarity with the architectural concept of the Lazaretto that existed, in my

---

[5] Adapted with permission from Griffith EEH: Angels and the Pandemic. *Psychiatric News*, May 2021. Copyright © 2021 American Psychiatric Association. All rights reserved.

boyhood Barbados, to isolate the individuals diagnosed with leprosy. It was a place not readily visible from the highway. Curiously, I never met anyone who spoke of having been on its inside. I could only imagine, even later as a physician, what might have gone on within this inscrutable place. Much later in my career, I learned the word *banishment* and its connection to these places.

It is hard now to remember how I got to the clinic in Saigon. A work colleague must have introduced me to the physician who ran the consultations. He may have invited me to stop by and make observations about his work. I entered the clinic. The doctor interrupted what he was doing and displayed the broadest and warmest of smiles. Then he presented me to his patient and gently urged us to shake hands. It was the strangest of experiences. The handshake was clearly meant to bring me and the patient together, to conflate our worlds and decrease his isolation. We were connected. I have always thought the doctor was insisting that I bear witness to the patient's humanity. The holding of hands, the welcome in it, now conjures up the famous line in the New Testament at Matthew, Chapter 26: "Now when Jesus was in Bethany, in the house of Simon the leper, …" One of COVID's first acts was to force interdiction of touching and assembly.

I never had the time to ferret out how that Vietnamese doctor came to be of such service, tending to the accursed in a country at war with itself and outsiders. I still see him amid this disease that so many years ago imposed the terror, isolation, and uncertainty that we have been living with for just a year. In an essay I wrote long ago, I referred to people who serve with such generosity as angels. Meeting them was a glorious experience.

## Welcome Happy Morning[6]

It was like a rushing wind. I crossed the threshold of a church's door on Easter Sunday this year and was met by a blast of joyfulness and hope. The noise of uncontrollable conversations. The rustle of paper. The to-and-fro of people undecided about where to sit. The crowd in the chancel placing chairs in a small and sacred space unaccustomed to the bustle. Different instruments and their owners invading where

---

[6] Adapted with permission from Griffith EEH: Welcome Happy Morning. *Psychiatric News*, June 2022. Copyright © 2022 American Psychiatric Association. All rights reserved.

only laity usually appear. Oh yes, it was joy in the morning. Even the program handed to me at the door signaled the change. I was surprised by the shine on its cover and the original artwork sprinkled throughout its 24 pages. On the front cover was emblazoned "You Are Welcome Here," and a quarter inch lower was the statement that masks are optional. In the center was a multicolored rendering of abstractions melded with the stone image of a cave. I could see inside because it appeared that the large stone blocking the entrance had been moved to the side.

What a contrast with the column I wrote in May 2020 and called "My Fable of Contagion." (The column appears earlier in this chapter.) I wrote then about the experience in another church at the time of the pandemic's appearance. I was preoccupied with the circumscribing of hope, the imminence of death, the upcoming isolation, and the short-circuiting of rituals that had long symbolized community. The experience this year was summed up in the very first hymn. It referred to life and health of all, vanquished darkness, sorrow ended, days of lengthening light, and bloom in every meadow.

As the time came for the sermon, I readied myself for the usual documentation of the resurrection. The rector surprised us all. He just walked up into the pulpit and declared that life was good. We ought to embrace it, as well as the people around us. It may, of course, only be my interpretation, but I think I heard him say that in loving and enjoying life, we make God's becoming man worth all the effort. The service ended with Charles-Marie Widor's organ piece, Toccata from Symphony No. 5, opus 42. Members of the congregation were crowded around the young organist, bearing witness to a resurgence of a community spirit and the resilience of an institution.

A week later, I attended a community-wide cherry blossom tree music festival in one of the city's parks (Figure 4.4). The day was sunny, with a brisk wind warm enough to encourage conversation and interaction through smiles and the occasional touch on the arm. One can always tell when people are relaxed in a park. The young families bring infants in prams and strollers. Spontaneous interchanges take place with minimal fuss. Police are generous, polite, and committed to helping the young, the old, and the disabled.

The musicians fit right in as well. It was evident that they had been invited with an eye on representing the community, to showcase diversity without fuss. I liked the group that played Bomba, the percussion-driven musical tradition from Puerto Rico. Conga drummers were present, as was a musician playing the Bomba barrel with sticks.

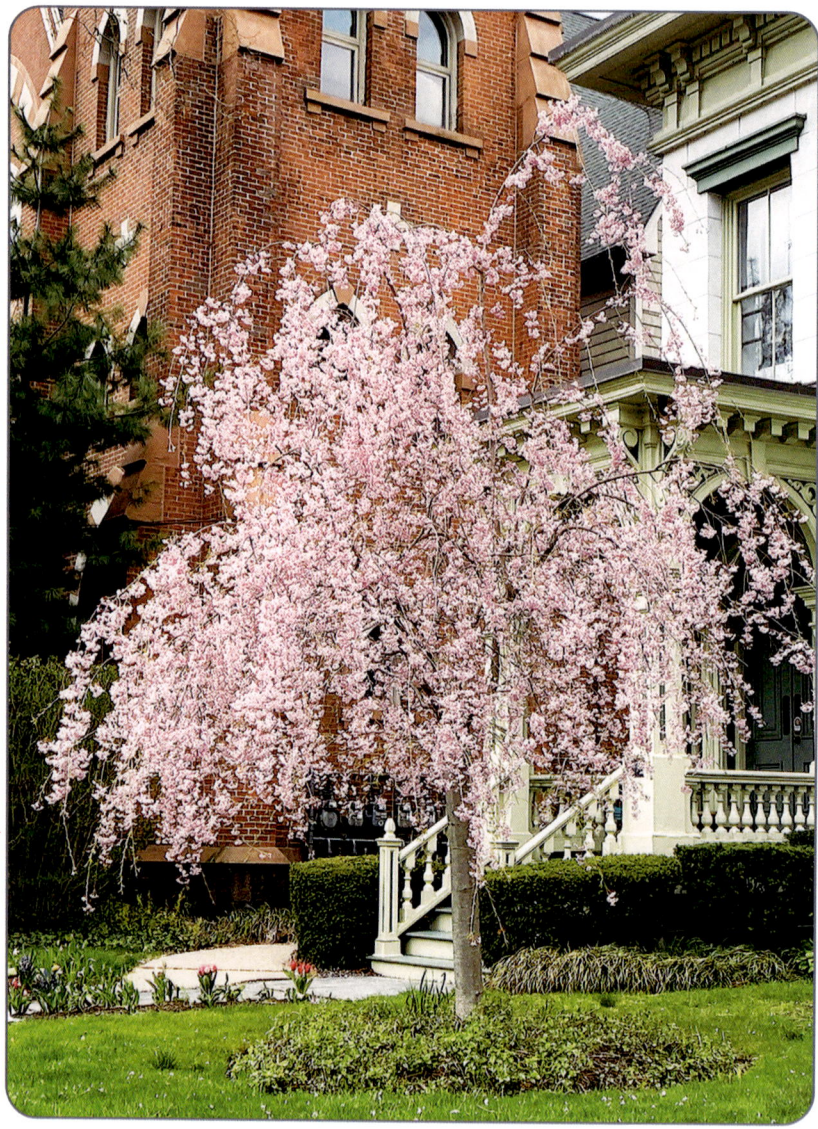

**Figure 4.4** Cherry Blossom Tree in New Haven, Connecticut.

Celebrating a spring cherry blossom festival while marking the weakening of the COVID-19 pandemic.

*Source.* Photograph by Brigitte Griffith.

A group of three women led the chanting. I recognized that an effort was being made to get past the fear and isolation imposed by the pandemic. I noticed that pizza was on sale, along with hot dogs and other finger foods. I laughed when I saw the long lines one had to endure to reach the food. Not a person complained that others were too close for comfort.

I learned that the cherry blossom celebration had been in existence since the early 1970s and had become a major afternoon event, except during the pandemic years. Cherry blossom viewing, I was told, is common in other cities across the country. It derives from a very old Japanese custom of aristocrats enjoying the viewing practice and finding inspiration for their poetry writing. This year, I marveled at the constellation of institutions marking in unique fashions their celebration of life. In my saunter through the park, I noted the most improbable backdrop: music and dancers jumping for joy, untroubled by the fact that they were moving to their own rhythms. They were out of step with the sounds emanating from the stage. Who cared? Everything one could see was a testament to health and life.

## Disguising War's Misery[7]

Military-type children's play was common in my long-ago Caribbean village. We imitated British-style army drills in my parents' yard, parading up and down with a designated leader. He would bring us to a halt, then present us to an officer who would carry out an inspection of our imagined uniforms. We knew somehow that military rank brought status and privilege, so no one wanted to be a private. We solved equity problems by rotating rank among members of the group, using caps from sweet-drink bottles to symbolize rank. We separated the cork from the metal covers and reinstalled them on the sleeve or shoulder of someone's shirt. We placed the round piece of cork on the inside of the cloth and into the cap that was on the outside. That way, everything stayed in place. Sleeve insignia indicated noncommissioned rank. Those with shoulder insignia had commissioned officer status, which mandated a salute before being addressed.

---

[7] Adapted with permission from Griffith EEH: Disguising War's Misery. *Psychiatric News,* January 2024. Copyright © 2024 American Psychiatric Association. All rights reserved.

Some of us had observed this marching at school among the older boys (and later, girls) who were members of the school's cadet corps. The upperclassmen were dressed in their cadet uniforms of khaki short pants and shirts, canvas belts with brass buckles, and berets. They marched to the cadence established by a corporal or sergeant putting down the "left, right … left, right … left, right, left." We saw the drills, too, on certain occasions at the Garrison Savannah, that wide open space that was a venue for special convocations. Members of the Barbados regiment and other paramilitary groups looked sharp in their crisp uniforms and polished boots. There could not have been even one young boy who did not at these moments dream of being a soldier. Later, I would see this form of military performance in Edinburgh, Scotland, at the famous Royal Military Tattoo. A similar hypnotic event takes place on Bastille Day (July 14) in Paris on the entrancing Champs Elysées when every branch of military and police march in splendor to public adoration. I believe that small and big countries put on these occasional displays to maintain this awe-inspiring connection between citizen and soldier. Military dress carries a message of sophisticated commitment to community citizenship.

I was drafted into the U.S. Army in 1964, a time when many young men contemplated the probability of ending up in South Vietnam in an unpopular war. I was assigned to a small public health unit and headed for Saigon. I was seconded to the Pasteur Institute to participate in research on bubonic plague, identifying rodent vectors carrying the fleas that spread the bacteria. I usually wore civilian clothes but often traveled in military vehicles and ate lunch in a building designated as a restaurant catering to the military. Vietcong occasionally lobbed grenades at such structures. They also tried to attach explosives to the underside of vehicles. It was a strange sort of life, different from the one led by friends who were seeing action in the countryside. Nevertheless, the unpredictability of attacks in the city, even though less frequent than elsewhere, still provoked an unpleasant and persistent anxiety.

I sat around on evenings in a community bungalow where I lived, listening to music from the Armed Forces radio station, chatting with mates, and writing letters. Irene Reid was one of my favorites then, a down-home jazz singer who kept my mind off war. Her song "That Bitter Earth" repeated "that bitter earth may not be that bitter after all." She offered some hope and asked, "What good is love that no one shares?" I wrapped my arms around my shoulders and prayed I would get back home safe. My other virtual soulmate was Etta James ("At last, my love has come along"). The music and quietness provided some comfort, even as they exaggerated the distance from home and made the risks to life more palpable.

I attended Sunday service in town at a church run by American missionaries. I joined the choir and was delighted to participate in the choral side of worship. Looking from the chancel area toward the congregation, I still see that man to my far left at the rear of the church sitting on a pile of hymnals. It took me a while to realize that he was on the lookout for any intruders seeking to lob a grenade or, worse still, penetrate the precincts of the church to do us harm. The pastor prayed so earnestly, seemingly oblivious to the war. I would look up and ask God whose side He was on. And I toyed with the idea of asking Him how He responded to the entreaties from the Vietnamese. I tried hard to comprehend the explanations offered by politicians back home to justify the killing and injuring. I never understood, after the departure of the French from Indochina, how the United States expected to win.

Ultimately, the parade ground, with its performative elements, and the war zone defy comparison. The aesthetic aspects of military dress uniforms and balletic parade-ground exercises are dramatic presentations focused on cadence, rhythm, and collective symmetry. Even when fighter planes fly overhead as a part of the presentation, they are in tight formation, representing some geometric figure finely held in check, leaving trails of multicolored smoke. No one dies on the parade ground. The horror show that is war takes place in another theater, displaying unspeakable suffering and unbridled hatred. The audience leaves the drama empty, pained, and marked by the performance. Others stay on the scene, permanently, as silent witnesses.

# Comments and Clinical Observations

I cannot stand up like a man, as they would say in long-ago Barbados, with my hands in pants pockets and leaning against a tree trunk or a neighbor's wall and state arrogantly that I was comfortable and at ease dealing with death and all its sequelae. It would not be the truth, even though, strangely enough, I did live in the shadow of death and dying while I served in the military. However, at that time and in that context, I did not think of death as a daily companion. I was not assigned to the combat front lines of the Vietnam War, repeatedly dodging incoming fire and keeping track of situations that might become the basis for future tales of bravery and manliness. I lived and worked mostly among the local population. Yes, I ran the risk of encountering an occasional grenade. However, members of my small preventive medicine outfit remained cautious and careful without being excessively preoccupied with the daily death toll on the front lines. I suppose my entire life may have taken a different turn if I had experienced sustained combat at the center of the hostilities and been forced regularly to contemplate dying for a cause that was always opaque and, to me, frankly unjustifiable.

I learned about death at a distance, through the common cultural ritual of the Protestant funeral service. I was a boy soprano for several years in the choir of the Anglican cathedral, in addition to singing weekly at one or two funeral services at the main cemetery chapel on the island. I had some understanding of the religious ceremony awaiting people at the end of their lives. I also had a precociously developed sense of what public mourning in Caribbean culture felt like.

As a young adolescent, I encountered the trauma of nature's unruliness. I witnessed Hurricane Janet batter Barbados in 1955 with torrential rain and wind. Houses resting on flimsy foundations took flight as though made of mere paper. Rivers overran their banks and floated chattel houses off their unstable foundations. Poles supporting streetlamps fell easily under pressure from the powerful gusts of wind. The pond in the back of my family home doubled its size in a few hours, and people knew to avoid its treachery, as it seemed angry. It was obviously deeper and no longer quiet, as it responded to the lashes of the gales changing direction constantly. Some people lost all that they had in that hurricane, including their lives. Fortunately, the terror of confronting the possibility of losing one's life was time limited, as it petered out in a day or so. I felt up close the adults' fear of dying, and I knew what it meant when they started praying audibly and with a certain repetitive intensity.

Amidst all the fear and suffering, I noticed another aspect of the turmoil. Neighbors helped one another solve practical problems: finding shelter for babies and for the aged who were bedridden; getting individuals to ground that was above the rivulets flowing in all directions; and avoiding contamination of food and potable water. The community came to life. The image of that public display of friendship stayed with me for many years. After the hurricane's departure, a sense of solidarity permeated the neighborhood. My eldest brother, a mere 17 years old at the time, was drafted to write letters to government officials describing the losses that neighbors had suffered. His missives served as testimonials that allowed neighbors to obtain money from the government for repairs to their property.

When the COVID-19 pandemic started in 2020, I was as thunderstruck as others, especially when the numbers of the dying started to increase. The Caribbean notion of being here today and gone tomorrow was on everyone's mind. Furthermore, international reporting indicated that religious organizations were being hit hard (Bacqué and Chemin 2020). That prompted immediate consideration of the relationship between man and God. Commentators worried about the pandemic's role as a punishment from above, and questions naturally arose about the gravity of our sins and their provocation of God's anger. The pandemic served single-handedly as a stimulus for my observation of life around me. And even now, I remain uncertain about my decision to title this chapter as representing an act of confronting the pandemic. For several reasons, one could claim that the coronavirus confronted us.

In my habit of perusing daily newspapers, I took notice of the virus's appearance, reported by Bacqué and Chemin (2020), among those who attended a large religious retreat that took place in Mulhouse, France. The account by Méjean and de Royer (2020) described the pandemic's effect on a group of Capuchin monks elsewhere in France. The connection between religious groups and the pandemic was firmly established in my mind because it was in church during my stay in Barbados that I first recognized the effect of the virus on daily goings-on. At a Sunday service, a priest mentioned changes in the administration of the Holy Eucharist, so that nobody could take a sip of wine from the common chalice. This administrative plan was followed days later by the abrupt closure of all churches, with no announcement of any date for a reopening. I left Barbados in March 2020 to return to the United States a few days before the international rules were put in place that restricted excursions over distance and gatherings into groups.

In the March 30 edition of *The New Yorker*, Jill Lepore (2020) published a historical review of plague, giving us a picture of what things were like in 1665 when the disease rampaged through London. She described how the British lost their bearings, and people prayed and screamed and sought help from any available source. Lepore's review was erudite and helped me understand some of the group phenomena that gradually materialized. Her analysis ranged across a wide landscape of what she called a "literature of contagion" before homing in on a discussion of the "plague novel." This review of the literature, both academic and mundane, made it even easier to structure observations of what was happening around me, to notice how others were constructing methods to pass the time, to dilute the anxiety, and to diminish the fear of tomorrow.

Some friends held prayer meetings by telephone several times a week. I inquired of a pastor how these prayer sessions were likely to be organized, and he taught me about prayer points. The first element would concentrate on giving thanks for several things: to medical personnel for their dedication to the task of caregiving and their willingness to expose themselves to the dangerous virus, to all those working to find a cure for the disease and preventive vaccines, and for the knowledge that despite everyone's fears God was ultimately in control of everything. In contrast to the focus on thanksgiving, the second phase of prayer would likely address the desires of those engaged in the praying: for the pandemic to end soon, for a quick return of pre-pandemic life, and for everyone to develop trust in the medical experts and their expertise. The pastor explained the importance of striking a posture in praying of being thankful without being demanding or boastful. Other community leaders encouraged the development of habits like exercising and taking long walks alone or with a trusted relative. I started music lessons on the steel pan with a teacher who taught remotely. I found the experience delightfully constructive and helpful in turning myself away from the negativity and bitterness that often accompanied the pervasive fear of the pandemic.

Later in 2020, I was hospitalized for a few days and felt the full impact of the pandemic's effects. However, I did not anticipate what enforced isolation in the hospital would feel like. I could receive no visitors. All personnel wore a mask, which meant that smiles, as a means of communication, had disappeared. When doctors came by to visit, they remained standing and at a distance. Friends told me stories about accompanying a sick relative to hospital and having to leave the patient at the entrance in the care of personnel, without knowing where their relative would be housed. On occasion, the patient was too sick to provide information easily. Consequently, family members felt like they had abandoned their relatives without being confident that the hospital admission had taken place smoothly. Obtaining information about patients became a difficult task in some cases, because hospital staff were justifiably cautious about giving patient information to someone who was inquiring by telephone and unfamiliar to staff. In my case, I could see that the nurses were working hard at being compassionate. Nevertheless, many of them seemed distracted by the existence of the virus and remained focused on respecting the rules that emphasized prevention of contagion. The accent was on isolation, distance, and reduced contact.

Some months later, I witnessed a patient's effort to gain admission to an outpatient clinic appointment accompanied by a relative. The refusal was emphatic. The explanation was that an immutable rule was in force denying entries by companions. Staff even explained that earlier in the week, a blind patient had tried to enter with a companion and was stopped at the entrance. Nurses recounted that story to underscore the rigidity of the rule and to make clear that its harshness was applied equitably. I was reminded of Jill Lepore's (2020) notion that serious pandemics tend to provoke brutality, even among caregivers who usually make liberal use of compassion.

Nicolas Truong (2020) wrote about a discussion with the French philosopher Claire Marin, which shed light on the basic idea that the pandemic was certain to cause ruptures in the social, professional, and family arenas. One objective of the pandemic was to fracture human connections. From that vantage point, my own observations took form and became more meaningful in time. Friends told me of adjusting to their closed churches by exploring services offered on television by different faith groups. They found it refreshing to hear a famous preacher from another part of the country. Technology was useful in that instance to bridge the gap created by distance. At the same time, some people obviously missed the distinctive pleasure of getting together "in His name." The professional disruption became a vibrant topic of discussion. To this date, the conversation continues about the merits of working from home compared with the positive aspects of coming together in the office. The pandemic reframed everyone's professional and home life. Some friends used the internet to attend art lectures offered by museums. These were wonderful ways to obey the rules that required us to stay at home while still engaging with the world outside our doorsteps.

The conversation between Nicolas Truong (2020) and Claire Marin warned us that technological advances might reduce geographic distance between us, but they could also augment the psychological distance. I suppose that induced me to take long walks outdoors periodically, with one friend at a time, both of us masked, savoring the unique pleasure of human contact. I mention these promenades also because many of us felt that the pandemic forced us to think about what was happening in the external world and to reflect studiously on the implications for different forms of human linkages. Apparently, several different strategies were available to confront the effect of stultifying isolation.

From these sessions of contemplation and reflection, some individuals derived ideas about being of service to others. I wondered whether the observable ubiquitous suffering, blended with the perceptible presence of death, forced a community-wide conversation about how to help others in the present context. Those who implemented efforts to assume the role of caregiver qualified for my categorization of being angels. Recognizing how the pandemic had disrupted routine life, I assumed that these angels imagined ways of calming the anxiety of others and themselves by providing companionship, reordering the home space to be less threatening, and focusing on stories that promoted nostalgia. The latter technique envisaged the possibility of seeing the beneficent and comforting landscapes of a pre-pandemic hometown or neighborhood. Many of us lived to bear witness to the arrival of that Easter morning service I described in the column titled "Welcome Happy Morning" (Griffith 2022). (This column also appears earlier in this chapter.) The churches were open again, and my rector entered the pulpit to emphasize loving and enjoying life. Later in that week so focused on resurrection and renewal, as I noted, people were outside, together, "conversating" as we would say back home, laughing, frolicking. Later, we would begin to think about what the future would look like. At that time, when the pandemic appeared to be waning, the cherry blossom trees in New Haven would make their appearance and inspire hope and promises of a new type of tomorrow.

Clinician colleagues told me of their experimentation with doing verbal treatments by telephone or by internet while the pandemic was in full swing. Necessity obviously required resorting to creative techniques. I had retired by the time the pandemic made its debut in 2020.

As a result, I was a mere witness to the reporting of discussions about the value of psychotherapy at a distance, the difference between audio evaluations and those done by audiovisual means. Claire Marin's predictions came to mind, as mental health professionals began to think about what they would keep or eliminate from their new ways of treating patients. I understood that similar discussions took place within hospital inpatient psychiatric services. Perhaps the most important reality was that the coronavirus had affected our lives and would leave us with a history of its passage. Numerous lives had been lost, some in an unceremonious fashion, with no leave-taking and no parting goodbyes. It was time to return to memories of self and others, of a past sense of security now trodden underfoot, and principles of patience, forgiveness, and love. No one was yet talking aggressively about setting up a we gatherin', a coming together that threw caution to the wind.

In reflecting on the pandemic in this chapter, I started by mentioning a Barbadian celebration called a gatherin'. The joy and hope engendered by this civic coming together were quickly extinguished by the pandemic's power and the ultimate frailty of human beings. We had no ready response to its blistering attack. The ensuing suffering affected us in one way or another. Many of us found someone, something, or an idea on which to lean and survive until we could say "Welcome happy morning." And yet, some of us are still in the throes of long COVID.

## Questions to Ponder

1. In your view, who is responsible for these recurrent, uncontrollable pandemics?
2. Do you consider the use of vaccinations in the struggle to control the pandemic a medical imperative or an optional political strategy?
3. Do you have a geographic space, real or imagined, usable for flights of restorative nostalgia?
4. The pandemic certainly left us with the notion that life constitutes an uncertain journey. How would you describe the elements on which you depend most?
5. Does de Chardin's notion of "Patient Trust" in God appeal to you?

## References

Bacqué R, Chemin A: Deux mille pèlerins, cinq jours de prière et un virus: à Mulhouse le scenario d'une contagion. Le Monde, March 27, 2020

Chawla D: Tracing home's habits: affective rhythms, in Stories of Home: Place, Identity, Exile. Edited by Chawla D, Jones SH. Lanham, MD, Lexington Books, 2015, pp 3–15

de Chardin PT: Patient trust, in Hearts on Fire: Praying With Jesuits. Edited by Harter M. Chicago, IL, Loyola Press, 2010, p 102

Dyer G: Existential inconvenience: life in the shadow of coronavirus. New Yorker, March 23, 2020

Griffith EEH: Welcome Happy Morning. Psychiatric News, June 2022

Griffith EEH: Race and Excellence: My Dialogue With Chester Pierce. Washington, DC, American Psychiatric Association Publishing, 2023

Josenhans FV (ed): Artists in Exile: Expressions of Loss and Hope. New Haven, CT, Yale University Art Gallery, 2017

Lepore J: What our contagion fables are really about. New Yorker, March 30, 2020

Méjean G, de Royer S: Coronavirus: les frères capucins du couvent de Crest fauchés par le mal. Le Monde, April 11, 2020

Truong N: Claire Marin: Il va falloir peut-être admettre que 2020 nous prépare douleureusement à l'idée de devoir vivre autrement. Le Monde, December 27, 2020

Walcott D: The Prodigal. New York, Farrar, Straus & Giroux, 2004

# 5

# Talking About Sacred Spaces

# Columns From *Psychiatric News*

## Healing at the Isenheim Altarpiece[1]

People have often called it one of the world's masterpieces, one with healing properties. Mathis Gothart Nithart, known as Grünewald, painted the panels of the Isenheim Altarpiece, and Nikolaus Hagenauer created its sculptures. The collective work stands in Colmar's Musée Unterlinden. Colmar is a small French city in Alsace, a region in northeast France. The altarpiece was built between 1512 and 1516 for the altar of the church in St. Anthony's monastery in the Alsatian village of Isenheim.

As Pantxika Béguerie-De Paepe and Magali Haas describe it in *The Isenheim Altarpiece* (2015) (Figure 5.1), the altarpiece takes on the structure of a polyptych with several hinged panels that close over a central section. The altarpiece provided pilgrims and other sick individuals readings about the Passion of Christ, the Annunciation, and the Last Judgment and stories about the life of Saint Anthony.

An early Christian mystic, St. Anthony reportedly lived on bread, salt, and water as a recluse in a desert hermitage until his death in the 4th century. Stories abound about his repeated struggles with Satan in the forms of dreams and visions. But Anthony eventually won the battle, augmenting his reputation as a healer and miracle worker (a thaumaturge). His name was linked to the healing of a severe chronic disease called St. Anthony's Fire. Anthonite hospices, such as the one at Isenheim established around 1300, are said to have concentrated on the care of patients with this and other skin diseases.

St. Anthony's Fire, also known as ergotism, resulted from eating bread tainted with a parasitic fungus that infected rye. Early signs of the disease were prickling and tingling of the limbs, which often progressed to severe burning pain, and necrotic tissue in the extremities. Convulsions, hallucinations, and pronounced pockmarks on the skin were said to be prominent symptoms of the illness. Béguerie-De Paepe and Haas (2015) described a ritual during which patients were taken in front of St. Anthony's image in the altarpiece and given a special drink in which relics of the saint had been dipped and containing plants

---

[1] Adapted with permission from Griffith EEH: Healing at the Isenheim Altarpiece. *Psychiatric News*, November 2019. Copyright © 2019 American Psychiatric Association. All rights reserved.

*Talking About Sacred Spaces*

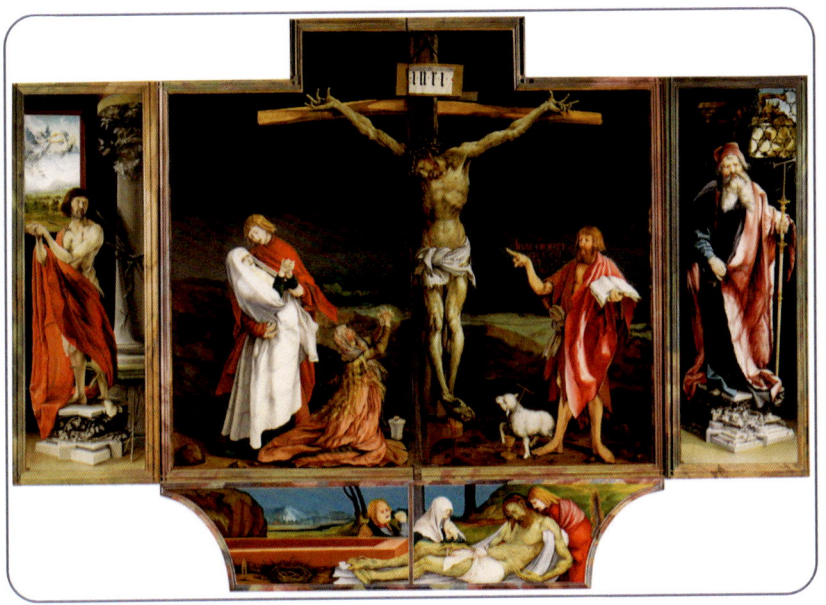

**Figure 5.1** A 16th-Century Altarpiece, Colmar, France.

Mathis Gothart Nithart, dit Grünewald. Retable d'Issenheim (fermé), vers 1512–1516. Colmar, Musée Unterlinden.

*Source.* Copyright © Musée Unterlinden/Le Réverbère.

with vasodilating or anesthetic properties. The caregivers also applied a balm to the skin. The disease was known for its morbidity and mortality.

The main panels of the altarpiece emphasize "suffering." Christ's crucified body is centrally positioned, with his head fallen on his chest and crowned with thorns. His body is thin and battered, marked and bloodied by soldiers' prodding. Béguerie-De Paepe and Haas suggest that this powerful image of the crucified Christ reminded pilgrims and patients, as they entered the Isenheim church, of the price of salvation and that their suffering was insignificant in comparison to what Christ had endured on the cross. The predella, the horizontal panel below the central one, shows Christ before he is entombed. The Virgin Mary's tears are visible. Mary Magdalene's eyes are red from weeping, and the crown of thorns sits on the floor. There is the image of St. Sebastian (known as a protector against plague) on the left panel and St. Anthony on the right panel. Their presence is justified because both were popular thaumaturgic saints. St. Anthony appears on other panels, indicating his honored status in this altarpiece.

Despite the marked suffering in the images of the altarpiece, I marveled at the therapeutic efforts of the caregivers in 16th-century Alsace. There was emphasis on the body's geography: the body's assaults, deterioration, and martyrdom—its ultimate loss of dignity. But what also shines through are the caring and uplifting of the human spirit, inspiring hope and nursing the suffering of others.

The effects of the disease were appreciated too well for there to be talk of a recovery movement. And so, the saints served their purpose. This was the early 1500s, remember. It was quite an experience for me to see this proof of an early healing community.

# The Steel Pan and Decolonizing Mental Health[2]

Just opposite my childhood home in Barbados, there was a shell of an unfinished wood house. Sometime in the early 1950s, a group of young men moved into the structure and started playing music at all hours of the day on empty, repurposed oil drums. The steel pan had made its appearance in my neighborhood. Trinidadians have always claimed the movement started on their island in the early 1900s. It was said to be connected to the earlier Tamboo-Bamboo musical groups from the era of enslavement. Once oil drums became available on the U.S. military base in Trinidad during World War II, experimentation with steel pans flowered. The modern pan then took root in the rest of the Caribbean, as a symbol of local creativity, and it now enjoys international popularity.

I witnessed its development up close in Barbados. The musicians practiced by purposeful repetition, picking note by note the tunes they wanted to learn. I recall the social stigmatization that marked the early players. While they bothered no one at all in the community, people saw them as a group of artists who enjoyed being out of work. As the years passed, their outsider status lessened and finally disappeared. Gradually, the steel pan movement invaded the island's schools and attracted girls and boys, men and women, old and young, and members of all social classes. The pan eventually appeared in every venue

---

[2] Adapted with permission from Griffith EEH: The Steel Pan and Decolonizing Mental Health. *Psychiatric News*, October 2020. Copyright © 2020 American Psychiatric Association. All rights reserved.

*Talking About Sacred Spaces*

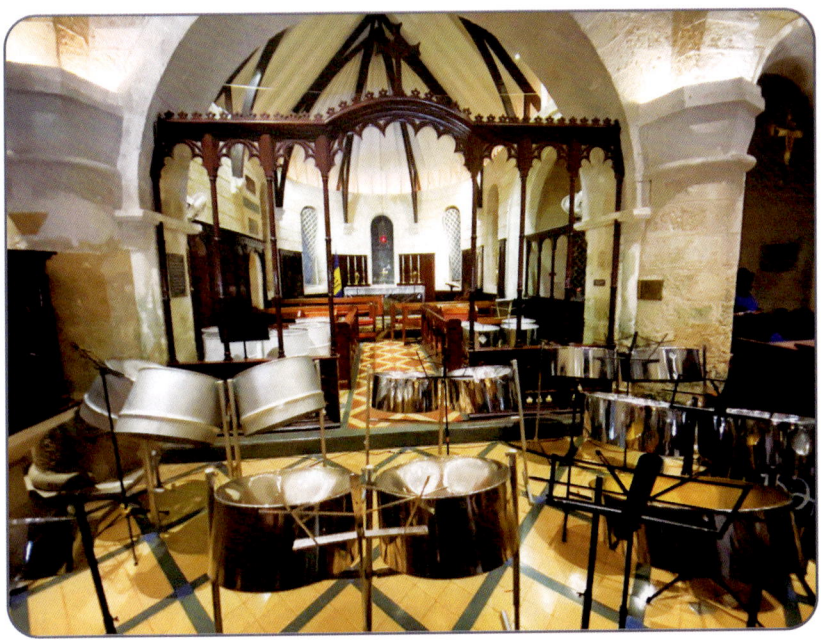

**Figure 5.2** Steel Pan Concert at St. James Parish Church, Barbados.

Steel pans of different sizes stand ready for a public church concert.

*Source.* Photograph by R. C. Grantham, AIA.

where Caribbean groups convened. The photograph (Figure 5.2) shows steel pans assembled for a church concert in early 2020.

My recent efforts to understand the pan as a postindependence Caribbean musical instrument have led to some intriguing findings. While it was used earlier to play calypso music and folk songs, artists are now using the pan differently. Earlier in the year, I attended a classical concert titled "Seasons in Steel." The program featured Vivaldi, Beethoven, Rossini, and Grieg, highlighting the connection between the steel pan and the composers' efforts to portray climate in their compositions. The musical results were impressive and illustrated the classical musicians' exploration of the European musical tradition with this indigenous instrument.

Some Caribbean cultural theorists have been urging the decolonization of Caribbean culture by cleansing local rituals and habits of European influence. In other words, they want the pan to serve as an anti-colonial symbol. However, these militants have met their match in the steel pan. They have not stopped its transformation into a powerful tool of creolization, present in secular and sacred music from Europe, the Caribbean, South America, North America, and Africa. The pan, not under any one group's control, stimulates freewheeling cultural interactions in social spaces.

Reports from experienced pan musicians suggest that learning to play pan has had a calming and soothing effect on some of their students, especially those who are hyperactive and showing difficulty concentrating. Some students in steel pan programs improve their academic performance and enjoy membership in music groups. Other pan players find the music important in making their environment beneficent, comfortable, homelike, and relaxing. Music makes them feel that they belong in a safe landscape. I enjoyed witnessing the use of the pan one evening to challenge the European colonizers and then on another night to promote local Caribbean tunes.

The pan seems almost to have a will of its own. It has enabled artists to refashion former geographies of painful colonial dominance into terrains of independence, sovereignty, and promise. It has contributed to the decolonization of the mental health sphere. I admire its thoughtful and expanded use by musicians who appreciate their professional freedom. Why not use the pan and adapt all kinds of music to it, employing it as a reliquary for rhythms developed at home and abroad? The point is to consolidate one's self-identity while rejecting subtle enslavement coming from any quarter. The steel pan artist, with this instrument and mallets in hand, is an important sociopolitical and psychological symbol. I hope the younger players develop a wide vision: one that surpasses the narrow boundaries defined by the tyrannical modern colonizers or the dictatorial descendants of the colonized.

# Peace Cranes in a Sanctuary[3]

Whenever I am away from home on Sunday, I find it rejuvenating to attend a church service as a visitor. I enjoy observing the rituals and listening to a new preacher. I take note of the level of the music ministry and the lay members' participation in their faith group. Most recently, I took the one-mile stroll from my lodging to St. John's Scottish

---

[3] Adapted with permission from Griffith EEH: Peace Cranes in a Sanctuary. *Psychiatric News*, November 2021. Copyright © 2021 American Psychiatric Association. All rights reserved.

Episcopal Church in downtown Edinburgh. I decided to visit this branch of Protestantism because I had already attended a service at a Church of Scotland, with its philosophy and rituals closer to those of John Knox and the Calvinist Reformers. One glance at the day's service program and my eyes landed on the claim that St. John's "seeks to be an open community, walking in the way of Jesus, engaging with an ever-changing world, and living a faith that is timeless yet contemporary, thoughtful, and compassionate." This declaration of modernity was in striking contrast with the graying mass of stone that characterized the external appearance of the building. The seeming contradiction would come up in my conversation after the service with the associate rector, the Rev. Rosie Addis.

Everyone followed the public health rules and wore a mask. The choristers took off theirs while fulfilling their duties, as did the clergy when leading the prayers, preaching, and reading the liturgical texts. Clergy and congregation had found an operational middle ground, a way of functioning while wearing masks and respecting distance. No collection plate was circulated during the service. A member explained that the new method, forced by COVID-19, was for someone to stand at the church door after the service, with the collection plate in hand. I learned that the new method is called "retiral collection."

It is hard to explain the Sunday morning peacefulness of an urban church, built almost 200 years ago. With the organ in the hands of an aficionado and the choir chanting the psalm expertly, the 16th-century motet by William Byrd was performed elegantly. The sacred sounds were bouncing lightly off the church walls, accompanied by the sun's rays dancing on the mobiles hanging from the ceiling and light fixtures around the church. The photograph (Figure 5.3) shows an example of the extensive mobile made of thousands of peace cranes handcrafted from origami paper. I learned the cranes were part of an exhibition by artist Janis Hart intended to transform St. John's Church into a bird sanctuary for peace. The idea was to provoke viewers into thoughts about the victims of the 1945 bombing of Hiroshima. That is complemented by the church's work for the inclusion of LGBTQ people in the life of the church and in society.

The Rev. Addis explained the mission of this urban faith group, first by helping me understand better the morning's sermon. It was about EFM, which stands for "Education for Ministry" or "Exploring Faith Ministry." She pointed out that this movement is not intended for the education of clergy. It is to help church members explore religious matters and facilitate their theological reflection about what God is asking

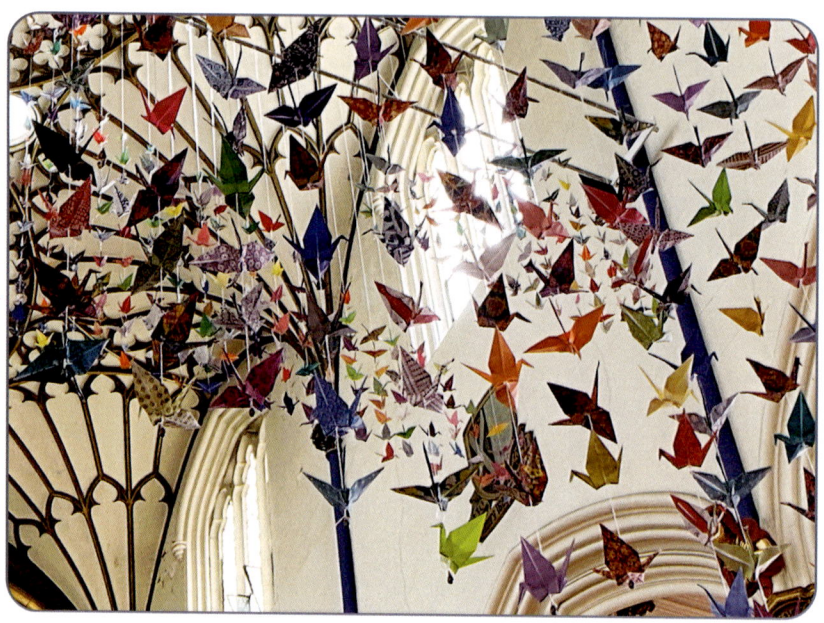

**Figure 5.3** Morning Church Service in Scotland.

A mobile of cranes floats above the sanctuary in St. John's Scottish Episcopal Church in Edinburgh, United Kingdom.

*Source.* Photograph by Brigitte Griffith. Used with permission of the Rev. Rosie Addis.

them to do in service to others. Hence the mission's orientation toward peace, abolition of nuclear weapons, and fellowship with nondominant groups such as Blacks, other minorities, and the LGBTQ community. Rev. Addis has also determined her pathway toward serving a unique group. She is an expert in British Sign Language and directs a monthly service for what she calls the "Messy Church." This meeting is for those suffering the indignities and problems related to hearing disabilities.

Several elements in the service collectively framed an ambience of togetherness and concern for others. The play area to one side of the sanctuary welcomed children. The tables and chairs at the rear invited attendees to socialize and enjoy tea and cake at the conclusion of the service. These ideas about caring for others, or for one another, reinforced the aesthetic and moral impact of the multicolored paper cranes fluttering in the air currents above us. The reminder of what we should do for neighbors was powerful.

# On Difference and Othering[4]

The Vocal Ensemble of the Choir of the Philharmonic Society of St. Petersburg, Russia, was featured in a Christmas concert last December in a Paris neighborhood church (Figure 5.4). Directed by Yulia Khutoretskaya, the ensemble performed chants from the Russian Orthodox liturgy and other traditional Christmas carols. They transported the audience on a trip to a different culture for the holiday season.

Russian church music is a genre full of deep rumbling bass and pure melodic tenor lines blending with the female operatic tones. The result in this case was a delicate harmony not always heard from singers who are all soloists. I have some familiarity with Russian church music, having sung with the Yale Russian Chorus during my early years at Yale University. In this performance, when the singers rearranged themselves in the chancel space while in full song with lighted candles

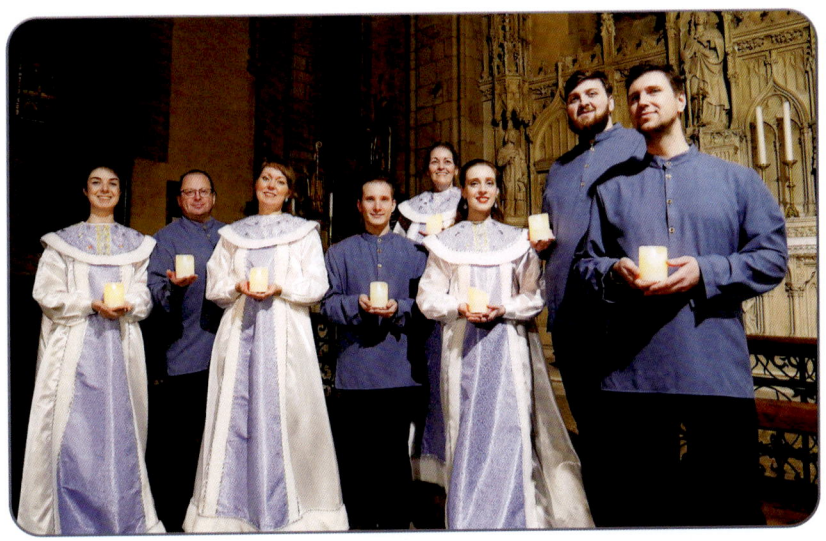

**Figure 5.4** Philharmonic Society of St. Petersburg, Russia.

This vocal ensemble, directed by Yulia Khutoretskaya, was known for its mastery of Russian liturgical music.

*Source.* Photograph by Pascal Belargent. Used with permission.

---

[4] Adapted with permission from Griffith EEH: On Difference and Othering. *Psychiatric News*, March 2022. Copyright © 2022 American Psychiatric Association. All rights reserved.

in the palms of their hands, the effect was magically breathtaking. The normally chilly church sanctuary became a warm cocoon.

Reflecting on my feelings during the performance of Russian music, I wondered why citizens of so many countries in the West have so little that is nice to say about Russia. I understand the differences in political opinion and approaches to economic theorizing. But are Russia's sins more egregious than ours? When we contemplate what we think is evil about them, have they surpassed the West? Is there nothing about Russia that could stir empathy in us?

The psychoanalyst D. G. Rao (2021) published a review of Isabel Wilkerson's book *Caste: The Origins of Our Discontents* (Random House, 2020). After exploring important ideas that tied Wilkerson's text to our social worlds, Rao described different factors that contribute to any caste system and distinguish "the high and the low, the privileged and the pariah" (2021, p. 414). He pointed out that there was something insidious about caste, with its established rituals and patterns that appear so naturally orderly. Rao eventually made connections between the mundane experiences in the social worlds affecting our psyches and their contributions to the creation and maintenance of caste structures around us.

An important mechanism that operates within caste structures is the presence of "othering" in what we do and think. Rao (2021, p. 419) called this universal tendency to "other" someone the act of "debasing, controlling, and dehumanizing" the other person. Rao separated "difference" from othering. Two people are different from each other along familiar axes that include age, gender, ethnicity, language, religion, disability, and other elements. Thus, difference "is usual, digestible, and can be celebrated" (Rao 2021, p. 419). However, when we extrapolate from difference to indicate inequality and inferiority, that is othering. The result becomes destructive and can lead to a withering exclusion of the other from social groups and community organizations. What strikes me, from time to time, is the ubiquitous nature of othering. It can be employed by individuals, groups, and nations. While we often use it reflexively, it can also be displayed with deadly intentionality.

I have followed recent news media reports of the dialogues between the leaders of the United States and Russia and find that they are remarkably similar in their logic, especially in their use of othering techniques. I realized, too, that we imitate these political leaders in the way we approach settling our differences with people we encounter in daily living. Staring at our competitors and seeing them as like us, just different along certain axes, require patience and endurance. It is convenient, but pointless, to view them as less than we are. That concert of Russian church music, even

*Talking About Sacred Spaces*

though I could not understand the language, still communicated a sense of the sacred and offered hope. It challenged the political leaders of both countries to cease the solipsistic bickering and recognize that othering one another is the way to breaking the peace. Recognizing mutual humanity is a better way to find common ground and avoid war.

## The Pleasure of Chance Encounters[5]

On a stroll around London, I found myself standing at the entrance to an aging Anglican church named St. Mary le Strand (Figure 5.5). The building I was admiring had been constructed in the early 1700s. I was fascinated by its location—it sat on a separate parcel of land in the

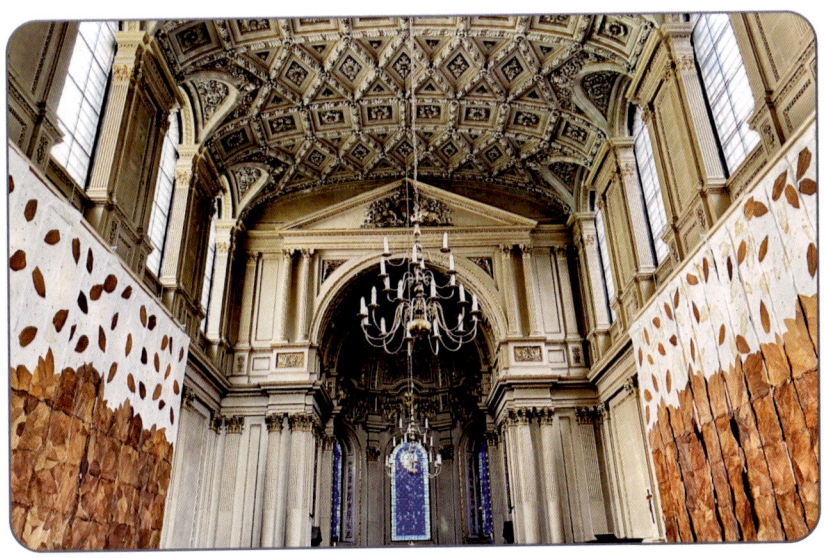

**Figure 5.5** Anglican Church of St. Mary Le Strand in London, United Kingdom.

This Anglican Church widened its mission to meet the needs of a mobile congregation.

*Source.* Photograph by Brigitte Griffith. Used with permission of the Rev. Dr. Peter Babington, Priest-in-Charge.

---

[5] Adapted with permission from Griffith EEH: The Pleasure of Chance Encounters. *Psychiatric News*, January 2023. Copyright © 2023 American Psychiatric Association. All rights reserved.

middle of a wide city street. Bustling life moved in all directions, while the edifice seemed unperturbed by the noisy modernity infringing on its boundaries. I have long thought it good for cities to have institutions in their midst that resist quietly the relentless march of footsteps. I noted, with some pleasure, that this church was unlocked and inviting passers-by to enter and visit its art exhibition.

The lady who greeted me encouraged me warmly to look around. And seeing my serious interest in the church and what went on there, she introduced me to the Priest-in-Charge, the Rev. Dr. Peter Babington. He explained that St. Mary was constructed on the Royal Processional Route that extends from the Palace of Westminster to the city of London and St. Paul's Cathedral. Located in Westminster along with the Houses of Parliament and Buckingham Palace, St. Mary has enjoyed the benefits of its geography. It has also been at the whims of developments affecting many institutions caught in the grips of increasing urban spread. Churches, particularly, feel the effects when congregants quit the city searching for a different kind of life. Those who remain behind sometimes worry that the burden is a bit heavier and the organizational mission more complex.

A slight despondency set in when I heard that for several years St. Mary had no full-time priest. In such circumstances, the expected community-wide debate was unavoidable—the one about whether the church should be closed. Fortunately, after the discussions, the Rev. Babington was invited in 2020 to take over as Priest-in-Charge. I imagined that the discussions touched on factors like those that confront civic leaders when a hospital closure comes up. Is there really a community need? Where will the financial support come from? Rev. Babington and I did not dwell much on these matters. However, he did articulate confidently the church's new tripartite mission: the church as a place of worship and prayer, the catalytic function of the church as a crucial link to other public institutions, and the cultural role of promoting and supporting efforts in the arena of arts and the humanities. Thinking about the hundreds of people I had seen moving around in the streets outside the building, it seemed obvious to me that having a sacred space in the vicinity was necessary.

The Rev. Babington was raised by his Anglican priest father and zoologist mother. After earning his undergraduate degree in applied chemistry, he worked as a chemist for about a year. However, he gradually recognized that both his faith and his life vocation were unsettled matters. After several years of contemplation and discussions with friends and advisers, he grew resolute about taking holy orders. He felt his decision to be ordained a priest was buttressed by an epiphanous coming to terms with a verse from the Gospel of Matthew 28:20: "Lo, I am with you always, even unto the end of the world" (King James Version). This prophetic promise of an eternal companion forecast his ordination to the priesthood in 1999. The promise also allowed him to counter my concern about the difficulty of visualizing God's presence while we are caught up in personal suffering. He pointed out that God does not intervene in our problems with our sense of immediacy. However, He is involved in His own way.

Besides our exchange about his pastoring to the community of St. Mary le Strand, we discussed the artistic collage of tobacco leaves installed on the sides of the sanctuary. Curated by Roberta Semeraro, "Conexión" is the creation of artist-architect Lidia León, who hails from the Dominican Republic. The exposition was a part of the 2019 Venice Art Biennale. Ms. León was raised in a family of Dominican tobacco farmers and is known for her involvement in social causes. She highlights the blending of Caribbean identities and the diversity of individuals' beginnings. The tobacco plants represent an important part of agriculture in the Dominican Republic and, in the present installation, are strikingly set against the architecture of St. Mary and the church's blue stained-glass windows. The photograph of the church's interior highlights this aspect of the sacred space.

I wish to emphasize the role that chance plays in these encounters. The view of people moving along different axes around the church in a busy street was a geometric puzzle. Within the building, there was this individual, obviously supported by others, trying to make the world a more beautiful and serene place. The light dancing on the suspended tobacco leaves contrasted with the more direct rays coming through the blue stained glass. Since that experience, I have seen the work of Henri Matisse, the modern French painter, who worked so intensely on enhancing the elegance of sacred buildings. There is an especial drive and insight that catalyze this creativity. Bearing witness to the imaginative, on an unplanned basis, is a wonder. It is more captivating than the usual museum visit.

# Exploring My Connections to Prague[6]

I could not believe my good fortune. I was strolling through Prague, the Czech Republic city I never thought I would visit. Several friends had told me that I would be stunned by the beauty of the Vltava River flowing under bridges and carrying along our hopes and memories. There would also be statues, ubiquitous churches, multiple squares filled with cafes and restaurants, and a variety of magnificent building facades and elegant doors. I was warned that once smitten, I would easily be pulled into a curiosity about Prague's place in the unfolding of history pertaining to the three regions of the Czech Republic: Bohemia, Moravia, and Silesia. However, I first had to revisit two probably surprising connections between Prague and me.

The first link came through my attending Sunday school during the 1950s at the Roebuck Street Moravian Church in Barbados. The Moravians benefited from the teachings of Jan Hus, a 14th- and 15th-century Czech theologian, Catholic priest, and philosopher. He became a Church reformer and important figure in the Bohemia Reformation. I visited the statue of Jan Hus that commands a major square in the Old Town region of Prague. Although executed in 1415 as a heretic by the Council of Constance, Hus's ideas lived on and led to the formation of the Hussite Church and broad religious, political, and social upheaval over several decades in Bohemia and Moravia.

The Hussites won several wars waged against them. However, they lost a battle in 1620 that caused a re-Catholicizing of the area. The Hussites also suffered from divisions within their own ranks, and the Unity of Brethren broke off around 1457. The Moravian Brethren, to avoid repeated persecution, received permission from Count Nicolas von Zinzendorf to start a new town and church in Herrnhut, Germany. They celebrated this renewal in 1727. Moravian missionaries arrived in Barbados in 1765 and are said to be the first missionaries who allowed the enslaved in their congregation. The Barbadian Moravian church that I attended was set up in 1834. Moravians contribute impressively to caring for the social, educational, and spiritual needs of the population. They taught me quite early about the task of caring for others.

---

[6] Adapted with permission from Griffith EEH: Exploring My Connections to Prague. *Psychiatric News*, August 2023. Copyright © 2023 American Psychiatric Association. All rights reserved.

My connection to Prague, this time more distinctly adult, relates to encounters with the work of Franz Kafka (1883–1924). Somewhere along my early university route, I confronted Kafka's books. Colleagues, more experienced than I in this sport of debating Kafka, suggest that the famous site in Prague, referred to commonly as "The Castle," is the source of Kafka's ruminations in his book. Having now personally toured the castle, I understand better that Kafka must have loved provoking his readers' imagination. The story of the man who arrived in town to take up a post in a famous castle is similarly provocative. There is repeated confirmation that for one or another reason he will not take up the post. The explanatory possibilities are legion. There may be a good rationale undergirding the man's rejection: he is a toy to be played with, those in charge are obsessed with their administrative power, it may be a simple lesson linked to the fundamental unfairness of life, or the author may have been contemplating his relationship with his father and an inattentive God.

Another of my interactions with Kafka (1915/2009) came through *The Metamorphosis*. The account of progressive deterioration and transformation of a human being into an insect was amplified when I read my colleague Michael Rowe's (2002) symbolic response in his text *The Book of Jesse*. Rowe described the experience of watching his son respond to the malignant effects of a progressive and incurable illness. His scholarly observations mirrored Kafka's catalogue of his subject's eventual loss of human dignity. Rowe meditated on how clinicians and family caregivers must fight against the temptation to abandon human beings caught in the distress of severe illness and bodily disintegration. It is at these times that the call for attention to the patient's humanity should be loudest.

A creative statue, by the Czech artist David Černý, celebrates Kafka in a nearby square. I found it a brilliant attempt to concretize in sculpture Kafka's literary expression of metamorphosis. Called *Kafka's Head*, it was erected in 2014, stands about 10.5 meters high, and weighs 39 tons (Figures 5.6 and 5.7). It is composed of 42 metallic sheets that move laterally and independently for 15 minutes each hour. The two accompanying photographs depict change produced in the appearance of the head.

My visit to the Kafka Museum required adjusting my eyes to its interior semidarkness. I tried to examine documents, listen to audiovisual reports about the author, and consider the objectives of the curated exposition. I learned that Kafka was sickly and did not have a long life. There was ample correspondence about his controlling and

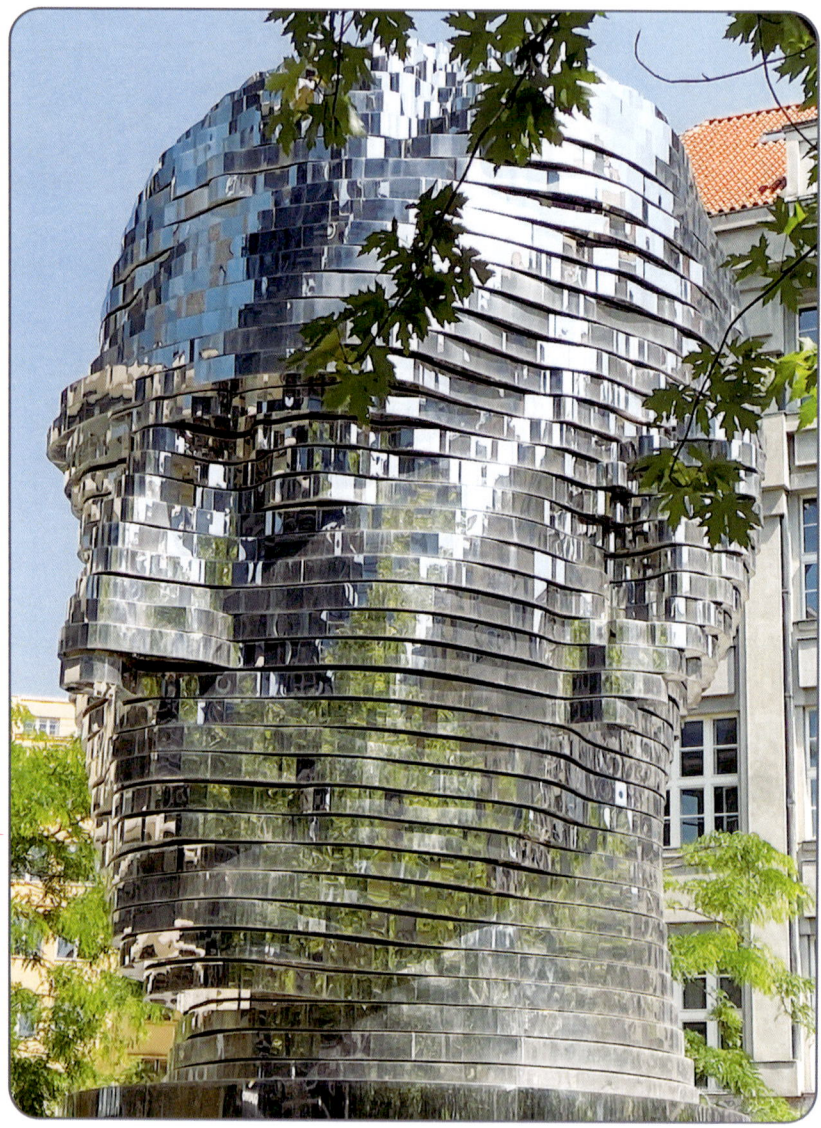

**Figure 5.6** Sculpture of Franz Kafka's Head by David Černý, Prague, Czech Republic.

This public twisting sculpture by a Czech artist captures the change in the appearance of the head as the 42 layers of metallic sheets are displaced as illustrated in this figure and Figure 5.7. The sheets move laterally and independently for 15 minutes each hour. At the end of this change process, the face returns to its normal structure.

*Source.* Photograph by Brigitte Griffith.

*Talking About Sacred Spaces* 137

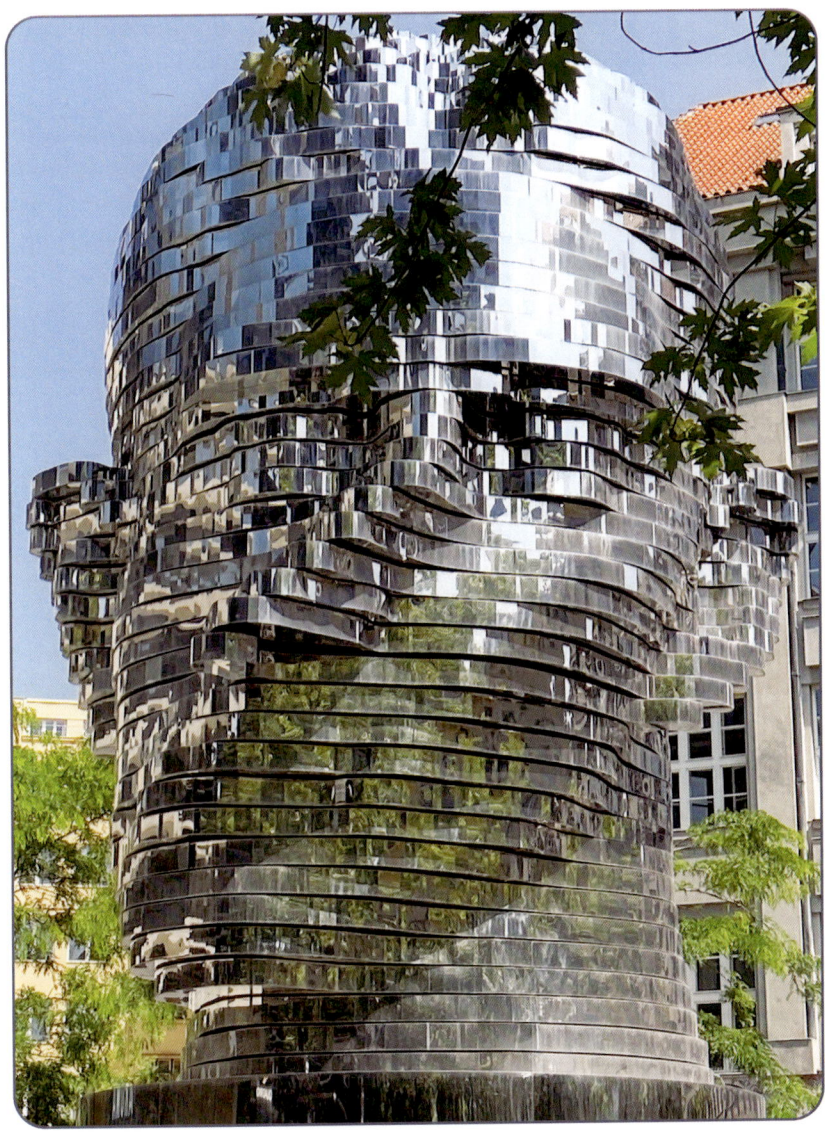

**Figure 5.7** Sculpture of Franz Kafka's Head by David Černý, Prague, Czech Republic.

This public twisting sculpture by a Czech artist captures the change in the appearance of the head as the 42 layers of metallic sheets are displaced as illustrated in this figure and Figure 5.6. The sheets move laterally and independently for 15 minutes each hour. At the end of this change process, the face returns to its normal structure.

*Source.*  Photograph by Brigitte Griffith.

authoritarian father, the constant poor health, the interactions with Jewish culture and religion, the inability to maintain solid connections with women, and the use of German in his work. I could feel his compulsion to write. I have come to appreciate his preoccupation with the absurdity of life, as Samuel Beckett and Jean-Paul Sartre take up in their own work. Kafka seemed to derive little pleasure from doing for others. The boredom in his existence was frighteningly palpable. Perhaps, he missed the Moravian call to serve others.

## A Migrant Amidst Mantuan Opulence[7]

Most of us have heard of the Italian city serving as an iconic symbol of high fashion, international sports, and world-class opera. Mantua, the English term for *Mantova*, located a mere couple of hours' travel from Milan, is set in another world altogether. The taxi I boarded at the train station took me to the middle of a beautiful city square called Piazza Erbe and left me to walk about 50 yards to the hotel registration desk. Once done, I ambled over to the hotel room set up in another building. I paused on the ground floor to watch a couple of sous-chefs make pasta from scratch. Later in the evening, I would taste what they were making, the lightly sweetened pumpkin dish called *tortelli di zucca*.

From my room balcony, I could easily survey the Piazza Erbe (Figure 5.8), which remains the site of a weekly city market. The restaurants and cafes that delimit the periphery of the square were illuminated by lighted table candles as the sun went down. They also served as a backdrop for pedestrians strolling by on the cobbled streets. I felt I was somewhere special. Its 2,000-year history and place on the list of World Heritage Sites convinced me I was visiting Mantua much too late in life. In high school back in Barbados, I had translated simple Latin passages of Virgil, the Mantuan poet. I had also come across Monteverdi's music in my choral experiences. All that had happened, however, without my making a connection to this city renowned for its art and culture. When I joined friends later for dinner, we could not stop talking about the magical ambience around us. The usual urban rush of traffic was gone, car horns silenced. Our only urgent concern was deciding which pasta to

---

[7] Adapted with permission from Griffith EEH: A Migrant Amidst of Mantuan Opulence. *Psychiatric News*, November 2023. Copyright © 2023 American Psychiatric Association. All rights reserved.

*Talking About Sacred Spaces*

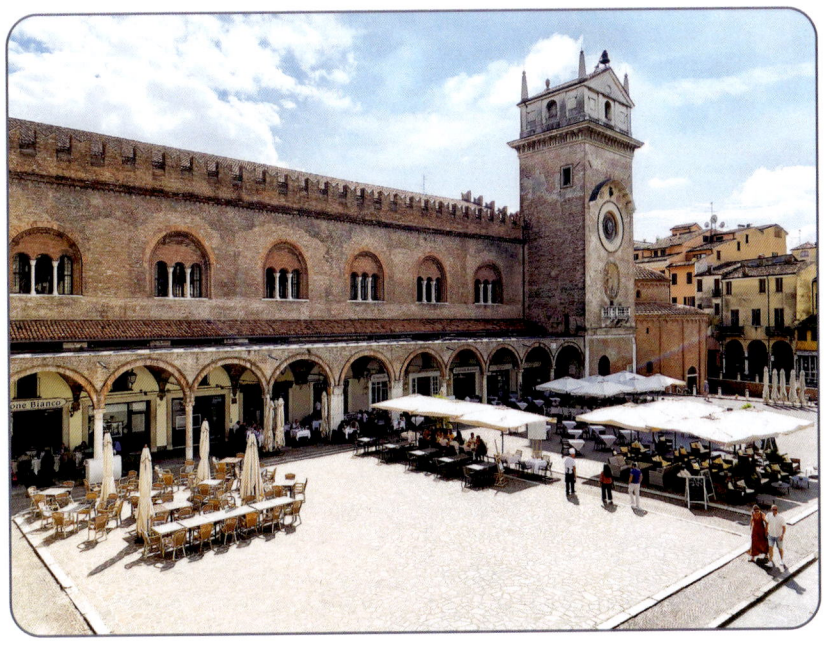

**Figure 5.8** Piazza Erbe in Mantua, Italy.

This Italian square has a 15th-century clock that marks the phases of the moon and signs of the zodiac.

*Source.* Photograph by Brigitte Griffith.

select. Fifty yards away, people held hands as they strolled around. There was a hushed quiet; people seemed to be loving life.

My tourist visits started with a promenade through the San Lorenzo Rotunda, an 11th-century circular church at one end of the city square. Across the street stood proudly the Basilica Sant'Andrea (Basilica of St. Andrew) (Figure 5.9), with its imposing steps. The grandeur of the church has made it an outstanding example of Renaissance architecture constructed between 1472 and 1765. The striking front façade of the church sets a contrast with the internal flooring of white and red marble arranged in a checkerboard fashion. There is a crypt, located below the magnificent dome and at the intersection of the basilica's nave and transept, that holds vessels said to contain the blood of Christ. Reportedly, the Roman soldier who pierced the side of Christ on the cross collected the blood and transported it to Mantua. The relic is exhibited in an annual street procession through the city on Good Friday.

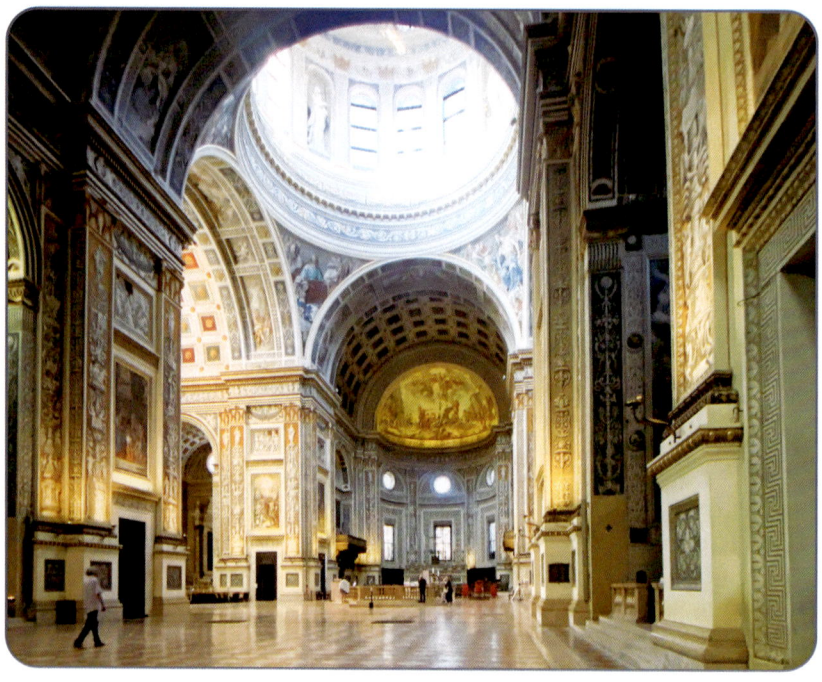

**Figure 5.9** Basilica of St. Andrew in Mantua, Italy.

The interior of this church is admired for its early Renaissance design.

*Source.* Photograph by R. C. Grantham, AIA.

The wondrous beauty of St. Andrew's Basilica made me think again about how much pomp and majesty are required for the execution of sincere religious rituals. I recognize the complexity of my own question, calling to mind a long-ago conversation with a member of a church. She explained that the poverty of her church's members could not stop them from finding different articles with which to decorate their church's altar. That special sacred space in their church had to "look pretty." It made them feel good and confident that their generosity toward the Almighty would be repaid. In our exchange, we never got to the problem of how much decoration is sufficient for the task of praising and pleasing God.

Another day on a morning walk, I was mulling over the historic dominance of the Gonzaga family, who were so influential in the Renaissance extension of Mantua and its artistic flowering. They had caused exceptional artwork to be produced in the family's palaces (the

*Talking About Sacred Spaces* 141

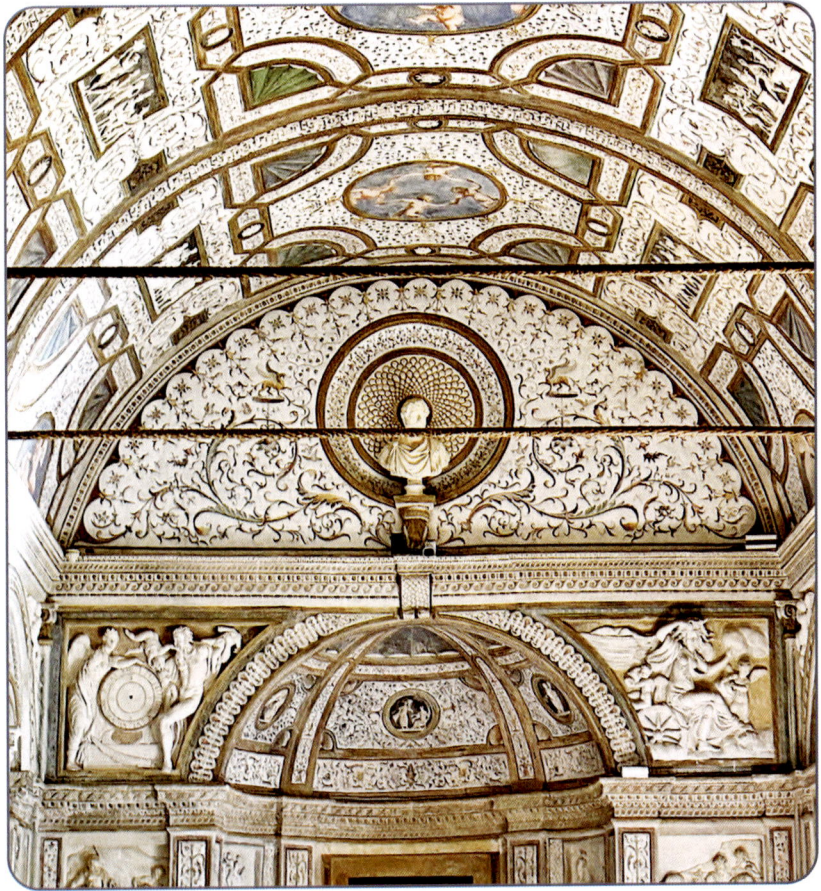

**Figure 5.10** The Ducal Palace in Mantua, Italy.

A photograph of the ceiling and doorway in a gallery of this world-famous palace.

*Source.* Photograph by Brigitte Griffith.

Palazzo Ducale and the Palazzo Te) (Figure 5.10). I encountered a young man who greeted me in halting Italian. For our mutual comfort, we soon switched to English. He asked for help to buy other food to supplement the bag of rice he was carrying. He was an African migrant who had come seeking employment, and he explained that although jobs were hard to come by, he hoped to find work soon. His hardship seemed to blight the value of the Gonzagas' contributions to the Italian patrimony. With the flamboyance of the Italian Renaissance, can we leave invisible the immigrant's plight in our midst? Is there a way for the financially disadvantaged among us to benefit from the Gonzaga beneficence?

Someone brought to my attention a report in Le Monde (September 25, 2023) written by Sarah Belouezzane and Gilles Rof (2023) ("L'Appel Vibrant du Pape en Faveur des Migrants"—"The Pope's Fervent Call on Behalf of Migrants"). On a recent visit to Marseille, France, the Pope seemed to respond directly to my reflections and concerns, making clear that the immigration problem is a major humanitarian and political quandary of the day. He recognized that seeking solutions with mere words is wasteful. People in the lower ranks of populations worldwide are seeking a better life, and that must be acknowledged. Underneath the search, which is sucking the life out of so many, is the quest for human dignity. This struggle, structured in modern terms by leaders of developed countries, makes clear that we must ask how may everybody benefit from the advances made by the upper echelons? Leaving the lower classes to fend for themselves is unacceptable and undignified. Many of us understand that action is required, of course. Still, implementing solutions in this era of polarized political convention is a major task.

## When Africa and Europe Meet in Church[8]

It was a glorious wintry day to stroll through New York City's Central Park, going from west to east, with a blinding sun warming the face. Solo pedestrians were carrying on telephone conversations with invisible others at the other end of the line. Nannies speaking foreign tongues pushed prams across the park as the motion and warmth lulled every baby into a lovable quiet. I was on my way to The Metropolitan Museum of Art (The Met) to follow up on a recommendation from an academic psychiatrist colleague that I visit the exhibition titled "Africa and Byzantium." He thought that the exposition might help clarify for me the community's initially negative response to the Spiritual Baptist Church's appearance in 1957 Barbados. My decades-long interest in this religious group is described in my book Ye Shall Dream (2010). Commentators have noted the movement's emphasis on liberation theology and improving members' self-esteem and independence of thought.

---

[8] Adapted with permission from Griffith EEH: When Africa and Europe Meet in Church. Psychiatric News, May 2024. Copyright © 2024 American Psychiatric Association. All rights reserved.

The historian C. M. Jacobs (1996) suggested that traces of the Spiritual Baptist faith appeared in Trinidad around 1815. He postulated that formerly enslaved Black Americans, who had fought on the side of the British in the War of 1812, were liberated and resettled in Trinidad. Referred to as "Merikun Baptists," they are said to have brought with them a Protestant Baptist liturgy. However, their worship style gradually included more ecstatic practices like dancing in the Spirit, loud singing and chanting accompanied by drums, bell ringing, blessing the church by pouring holy water at the four corners of the edifice, and getting into the Spirit at the center pole of the church. Colonial government authorities were apparently concerned that this style of Africanized practice might undermine the spread of Christianity. The church group, finally labeled Shouters and disturbers of the peace, was outlawed in 1917 and regained legal status in 1951. That decision followed considerable political debate within the Trinidad legislature.

Nourishing his church in Barbados during the late 1950s, Leader Granville Williams maintained the practices that he had learned from the Trinidadians. These ritual elements evoked antecedents of African worship, particularly since they were unknown to other church groups in Barbados. Many Barbadians felt that the "Africanities" pointed in the direction of the dark arts, and they concluded that the novel practices were a throwback to the 1940s and 1950s. That was when common talk of Obeah tales frightened children and others who feared being hexed. However, Williams made clear from the start that his activities were grounded in his connections to the Holy Spirit. There was no linkage to African deities and rituals that one might see in Caribbean Shango, Espiritismo, Santeria, or Vodun. Still, the Barbados Spiritual Baptist group encountered community opposition related to theology. Nonmembers obviously thought about what had occurred in Trinidad, while converts to the new faith insisted that they were centered on Christ. Believing in Jesus and walking in His ways led to the acquisition of powers of foresight, healing, and an ability to communicate with the spiritual world of angels and saints.

Between the 1950s and 1980s, there was also much discussion on the island about Black power, Caribbean independence, a renewed interest in Africa, and a growing intolerance of White privilege. The Spiritual Baptists talked about Blackness and its links to economics, politics, and music, while also insisting that Jesus was a Black man. One would have thought that this secular turn to Black politics and culture would have been neatly melded with the rearrangement in religious ethos. Instead, the Spiritual Baptists were taunted and mocked, and their head ties were publicly pulled apart. Of course, time gradually healed this type of disdain, and the public attenuated its own criticism and grew tolerant and even friendly.

As the years passed, I wondered about the difference between community objections to the arrivals of this new movement and a deeper, but quieter undermining by the older established churches on the island. The latter conveyed a feeling that African culture knew little about the Christianity of the European-grounded missionary churches. However, in my visit to The Met, I realized that Africa had seen Christianity up close for a long time between the 3rd and 7th centuries after Christ. St. Mark reportedly brought the religion to Egypt in 49 C.E. By the 4th century, Christian communities in Egypt were flourishing, and Eritrea and Ethiopia had formally adopted Christianity. Here I was, looking at a 6th-century Egyptian wool tapestry depicting Mary holding the infant Christ and the archangels Michael and Gabriel at her sides. There was also in the exhibition a wall painting from 10th-century Sudan of a bishop being protected by St. Peter. All of this predated the work of Portuguese and Spanish missionaries between the 15th and 18th centuries who spread Christianity along coastal Africa.

It seems clearer now that the Spiritual Baptist message of melding politics and theology was initially too complicated for the colonizing churches and their conservative congregations. Acceptance of the religion has improved in recent decades, although I have not observed much enthusiasm for the notion that Jesus was Black. In any event, The Met assured me that Africa was not as impervious to Christianity as some assert. While being politically anti-colonial and against White privilege, Williams saw Christ and the power of the Holy Spirit as a powerful tool to combat colonial oppression. He wanted to frighten Whites, not Blacks, with the power to heal and to talk with the saints.

*Talking About Sacred Spaces*

# Comments and Clinical Observations

Sacred spaces have long occupied my attention, perhaps because they were central to my childhood activities as early as I can remember. In recent discussions with a longtime Barbadian friend, we enjoyed our recollections of attending 9:00 A.M. Sunday school at the same Moravian church, then going off to matins at different Anglican churches. Methodist churches had Sunday school in the afternoon, and Anglican churches had 7:00 P.M. services, where both of us sang in choirs. These were our Sunday habits for many of our youthful years, which were eventually broken by the act of migration: he to London and I to New York. In Barbados, our repetitious routines were solidly reinforced by parental demands and traditions. Sunday was church day! The presence of formal sacred spaces in our two lives was so natural that attendance in church became a practiced habit long before we realized it.

In our conversation, my friend and I came almost simultaneously to the conclusion that there was no other permissible choice. Even if, for example, we had met the extremely high bar of finding an acceptable excuse for not going to church, we still could not have played outdoors or made noise for neighbors to hear. In 1950s Barbados, in our two villages, Black children went to church. No one cared which faith group you chose. That was a personal choice made by parents or their surrogates. My friend noted that even whistling was not permitted in his home on Sundays. Such an act contravened God's law. It would also have been taken as a sign that he was claiming manhood and asserting a bit more autonomy than the adults were disposed to accord him. He, and I, had to go to church, which turned out to be pleasant enough because friends were hanging out in that landscape. In any case, staying home on a Sunday was to confine oneself to a day of boredom, practical immobility, and imposed solitude. I am sure that much of that has now changed, with Sunday being a day often used for organized football and cricket matches, picnics at the seaside, and trips to the countryside for lunch. The island's emphasis on tourism has forced use of Sundays for a broader spectrum of activity these days. That is in addition to the expansion of other religious groups' use of Saturday, instead of Sunday, as their day of worship.

It took me many years to appreciate the contributions that religious institutions made to the daily rhythms of life in secular spheres. The art of reading, writing, and speaking were all influenced by church practices. So were sensibilities related to fairness, honesty, and justice. Two key notions that became important in my academic life, dignity and love of narrative, clearly had roots in church. The other force was my early encounter with different forms of church music: the chanting of psalms in the Anglican tradition, the fast-tempo songs of the Pentecostal movement used to facilitate the arrival of the Holy Spirit, and the dirgelike chants my mother used as a tranquilizer to right her mood at home. As I said, church music in my boyhood was a potent force. In adulthood, I realized that my friends from back home and I had committed to memory many psalms and hymns, innumerable stories from both Old and New Testaments, Christmas carols, and even liturgies for weddings and funerals.

A few weeks ago, I heard a story that involved my father. A Barbadian orchestra was playing at a dance taking place in a New York City church basement. The band started to play a popular tune we all recognized as a hymn, but in calypso up-tempo style. My father told the musicians that they should not have transposed a sacred hymn into a jump-up piece. The band stopped playing it. The habits of sacred spaces can, in some communities, keep us close to what the community feels is good and spiritual and respectful of certain secular traditions. These are the aesthetic practices of the cultural anthropologists. In highlighting this potential strength of the sacred space, I am not denying other weaknesses or potential misuses of faith communities. However, those stories are worth exploring later. I go on here to point out that in the vignette I just recounted, some readers may readily see the tableau representing an act of resistance by Barbadian youths against the music some may view as symbolic of colonization by White European missionaries.

In yesteryear's Barbadian village, the communal understanding was that one went to church dressed neatly. I am aware that such imperatives have lost their influence, especially in urban communities. These days, churchgoers present themselves all over Barbados both dressed up and dressed down. And one can find the same breadth of fashion in New York, Paris, and London. But once upon a time in their Sunday deportment, Barbadians reflected the church's subtle and almost invisible emphasis on the notion of dignity. In my village, even the poorest family found a way to make sure that children attended Sunday school looking cared for. At a minimum, this meant in clothes washed and pressed and with hair combed. If observant, one would notice how mothers were informed about the techniques for keeping Black skin looking healthy and not shiny and full of infected bites from sandflies and mosquitoes. In Sunday school, one could also observe mothers' attention to their young daughters' coiffure and general aesthetics.

I believe it worth reminding readers about the centrality of sacred spaces in communities where money is not abundant and income not easily or readily disposable for leisure activities. I first participated in theater and in choral singing organized by a church. Friends of mine represented their church in soccer and in scouting. When these community activities become popular among youths, they may expand rapidly, especially in geographic areas where financial resources are abundant.

Some churches offer vocational classes where members learn a trade, clinics that cater to those with medical and psychiatric needs, academic classes at different levels, and groups that discuss current sociopolitical topics and church history. In addition, some faith groups have taken a special interest in refugees, the homeless, and individuals with unusual disabilities. When I first arrived in New York City in 1956, I accompanied my father to a Harlem church that supported the theater arts. It was also when I first heard of Black pastors who were vibrantly active in politics and used their congregations to influence outcomes of elections. In time I would understand that sacred spaces could be transformed into loci for the molding of identities and the formation of voting groups committed to identity politics.

In my wanderings, I have been struck by certain other developments I have encountered in recent years. First is the preoccupation with different forms of a healing ministry: caring for people with alcohol and drug use or discussing formally the principles of biblical healing. Second is the turn to a renewed interest of churches in providing housing to the needy. Finally, there seems to be a recommitment of these organizations to offer feeding programs.

I remember clearly a conversation that took place in New Haven, Connecticut, at the time I was director of a major clinical unit at the Yale School of Medicine. I was involved in outreach activities beyond the medical school arena, and I engaged regularly in discussions with community activists. One day, I was earnestly engaged in some political strategizing, seeking an alliance with a group of pastors. One of them, popular and highly respected, asked me why his group should be involved with my program. He pointed out that his major mission was to care for his parishioners' souls. I decided that he had to be testing me. He could not simply be so unaware of all that the Black church had done over the years in health, education, politics, and just the overall promotion of general well-being of Black people. My answer was fluent and unwavering because I cited numerous examples of all that the Black church had done for their communities. I did not attack him. I simply extolled the creativity and hard work of Black church leaders in a social and political sense. That included their activities in confronting substance abuse, contending with homelessness through leadership of housing solutions, and catering to preschoolers in special programs. I had to believe that he was impressed by my awareness of the importance of sacred spaces in all communities. I pointed out that caring for their souls had a futuristic tinge to it, and Black bodies and minds deserved ongoing attention. He said little after that. The group of pastors supported my outreach efforts for years.

Looking back at my columns, I recognize the breadth and variability that are visible and palpable concerning the involvement of sacred spaces with healing of individuals' bodies and minds. The Isenheim Altarpiece makes clear how churches were involved with travelers and their suffering and the presence of incurable diseases that afflicted everyone but devastated the poor. In the column about the steel pan, the church welcomed this indigenous instrument into its midst and helped dilute the social stigma attached to its non-European origins. Because of their expansive spaces, church buildings also can afford to provide practice venues for the large steel drums. The Scottish church I mentioned used its sanctuary to promote art, with its visual and psychological effect, while also promoting peace and highlighting the clinical needs of the LGBTQ community. Also, a community church in France developed the musical program that brings a choir specialized in Russian liturgical music to celebrate Christmas. This facilitated reflection on the fundamental characteristics that separate the concept of "difference" from the practice of "othering," which we use to malign those who are unlike us in some way. Finally, the column on Mantua raises questions about the tendency, of those who lead certain sacred spaces blessed with wealth and fame, to ignore their needy neighbors.

Another column, focused on the encounter between Africa and Europe in church, describes the confrontation between European theology and praxis as it met the cultural terrain of Africa in places like colonized Barbados. This is a phenomenon that has plagued colonized spaces for many years. This interaction of different religious beliefs and practices in the context of colonization is manifest in the indigenous development of the Spiritual Baptist Church throughout the English-speaking Caribbean. People like Archbishop Granville Williams, who founded the Spiritual Baptists in Barbados (Griffith 2010), regularly interrogated observers with questions focused on the interactions of local populations with their White colonizers. Why did White persons suggest or imply that Jesus was White? Why did they hide the power of the Holy Spirit from Black people? Why were we kept poor? Why did the oppressor White people insist that we follow their religious practices? Why did they worry so much about the joyful, rhythmic aspects of our traditions, which reflect our cultural heritage? And why did they use so much effort in rendering opaque their efforts to colonize Indigenous populations?

In commenting about my early interactions with Barbadian faith groups, I mentioned only Protestant churches, which exclusively defined my personal experience. In the 1950s, the Anglican Church and its Protestant derivatives (e.g., Methodist, Moravian, Brethren) dominated the church scene. Since that time, Catholic and several other Protestant groups, as well as an influx of Muslims, have multiplied their presence and influence. This evolution in the range of sacred spaces reflects the history and sociopolitical changes within each Caribbean island. This includes whether local governments supported their religious institutions economically and politically.

I promised to return to the important notion that sacred spaces have never been consistently beneficent for all users. In other words, churches, synagogues, mosques, and other sacred places may, from time to time, be perceived by their users as hostile environments. I expect this is true about many institutions that serve large communities, such as political parties, universities, social groups, military outfits, and medical groups. Sacred spaces can deteriorate through the corruption of their charismatic leaders and by subgroups within the membership seeking to promote personal interests. There is no need to reemphasize here the wars and violence that characterized the reforming of church ideologies over the years. Many of us are familiar with religious groups' current discrimination against women and LGBTQ groups. We know, too, how organized religion has promoted exploitation of some subgroups. Indeed, many scholars have claimed that sociopolitical colonization has frequently been accompanied by the emphatic presence of clergy from one faith group or another. I expect most of us hope that it is much easier to highlight the positive elements of these religious organizations than to catalogue their transgressions. My thoughtful, meditative friends repeatedly assure me that human beings who lead and direct these organizations always bring into sacred spaces the problematic aspects of their humanness. Recent stories of the torment in the Anglican Church of Great Britain illustrate this dilemma. Ducourtieux (2024) described the extent of several scandals in this branch of Anglicanism that have been serious enough to provoke resignation of leadership because they apparently ignored the existence of problems among clergy and others. These events are inevitable, I am told, and I must not give up faith that these institutions are fundamentally worthwhile. The work within sacred spaces always includes efforts to purify the air and to differentiate between the organization and its members.

Before leaving this chapter, I must linger in discussion of a peculiar feeling I have especially when I am visiting an area overseas that is unfamiliar to me. I may be disquieted for some reason, somewhat anxious, and looking around for landmarks to minimize my confusion about where I am. The sight of a church is calming. If I enter the church at that time, I am immediately distracted and curious about its architecture and wondering about the individuals around me and what their requests of God may be. The surroundings, especially in neighborhood churches, are generally quiet and give the impression that they are being used for solace and to restore a certain equanimity of spirit. In Romania a few years ago, citizens who entered the churches I visited immediately looked for the statues of saints and kissed them while making the sign of the cross. These visitors seemed relieved to be inside a church in the middle of the day. Sitting inside the sanctuary, with daylight shining through the multicolored windows, has always been a form of respite for me.

The pastor was trying to provide this experience in that busy area of London, called Westminster, where passers-by were hurrying in all directions. St. Mary le Strand was offering the additional pleasure of an art show on the interior walls of the sanctuary. This was creation of a space for repose and calm, a sort of home space considered safe, quiet, devoid of conflict, and able to facilitate recuperation from fatigue.

When I visited that London church, I remember being welcomed by a gracious lady who offered me coffee and made me feel welcome to sit and observe the art exposition. I was encouraged to pose questions about the edifice and its mission. This was an effort to ascribe dignity to our transaction and to make me feel at home in church. The experience reminded me of one time when I visited a church during midweek and found that an organ concert was in progress. It was a joyful and transcendent moment.

## Questions to Ponder

1. Are you now able to list 10 roles that are considered a part of the mission of faith groups you know?
2. What do you consider the two most important roles of faith groups?
3. Should sacred spaces be protected by governments?
4. Should clinicians encourage their patients to make use of sacred spaces?
5. Do you regularly ask people about their personal or family commitment to the use of sacred spaces? Does this information tell you something important about them?

## References

Béguerie-De Paepe P, Haas M: The Isenheim Altarpiece—2015. Colmar, France, Art Lys, 2015

Belouezzane S, Rof G: L'appel vibrant du Pape en faveur des migrants. Le Monde, September 25, 2023

Ducourtieux C: L'Église d'Angleterre dans la tourmente. Le Monde, December 27, 2024

Griffith EEH: Ye Shall Dream: Patriarch Granville Williams and the Barbados Spiritual Baptists. Kingston, Jamaica, University of the West Indies Press, 2010

Jacobs CM: Joy Comes in the Morning: Elton George Griffith and the Shouter Baptists. Port of Spain, Trinidad, Caribbean Historical Society, 1996

Kafka F: The Metamorphosis (1915). Translated by Wyllie D. Cabin John, MD, Wildside Press, 2009

Rao DG: Book review of Caste: The Origins of Our Discontents by I Wilkerson. J Am Psychoanal Assoc 69(2):412–421, 2021

Rowe M: The Book of Jesse: A Story of Youth, Illness, and Medicine. Washington, DC, Francis Press, 2002

# 6

# Focusing on Place

# Columns From *Psychiatric News*

## Celebrating Psychiatric Health and Place[1]

I offer several examples to illustrate that "geography" has become increasingly connected to both general and psychiatric health. The Nobel Laureate Derek Walcott (2004) described his search for home, with tropical St. Lucia as his reference point. There, sunlight and sea transformed his body and made it sing and hum. Mindy Fullilove (2004), a professor of urban policy and health at the New School for Public Engagement, described how the bulldozing of a city's neighborhoods produced stress reactions in people who had lost their homes in such brutalizing urban renewal. Michael Rowe (2015), a Yale professor and mental health theorist, has explored what factors enhance or impede the successful reintegration of severely mentally ill patients into their home communities after an acute phase of illness. Some of those factors are intrapsychic and others environmental. All are related to the patients' regaining the skills to return to the rights and privileges of community citizenship.

"Geography" represents the construct of place, space, landscape, or terrain. In recent years, medical anthropology and medical geography have taken the lead in the relevant scholarship that clarifies the interaction of place and both general medical and psychiatric health. It is accepted that the idea of a healing environment encompasses the physical dimensions of the space as well as the enactments and rituals related to biomedicine that take place within the space. That is why home-space becomes a healing environment when family members participate meaningfully in their caregiving roles. As I noted in the previous chapter, many religious groups are currently expanding their remit and redefining their commitment to becoming healing communities.

I visited a recent exhibition titled "Personal Geographies" at the Yale Center for British Art. The focus was the English painter Eileen Hogan (born 1946), whose work combines attention to portraits and landscapes. Her visual presentations captured individuals interacting with their unique spaces. It was left to the viewer to divine the quality

---

[1] Adapted with permission from Griffith EEH: Celebrating Psychiatric Health and Place. *Psychiatric News*, July 2019. Copyright © 2019 American Psychiatric Association. All rights reserved.

of the interaction between these two fundamental elements. For example, one portrait revealed Britain's Prince of Wales, without necktie, sitting at his desk in a naturalistic, informal home setting, attending to correspondence. Conveying measured relaxation and a modicum of task-oriented activity, it illustrated the therapeutic aspects of limited work or active leisure.

Hogan also spent time painting unique dimensions of public parks in Britain. In commentary on the exhibition, she explained that she had sought opinions from the public about their preferred park areas. So, for example, she painted an intimate and personal pathway surrounded by lush greenery; on another canvas, she highlighted the simple gushing of silvery water from a 3-foot-high sprinkler. Both scenes evoked images of nature catalyzing reverie and healing calm. Art critic Kathy Czepiel (2019) explained that "Hogan's ability helps us see places and people both as they are and in a new light."

These thoughts reminded me of my attraction to the Danielle-Mitterrand garden (Figure 6.1) in Rue de Bièvre, a narrow street located in Paris's 5th arrondissement. This tiny park, named after the wife of a French president, offers a tranquil space away from mundane pressure to rest, recuperate, and think about those whom one loves. I don't wield a paintbrush of any sort. But there, I have wondered at the magical effect of the architect's and urban planner's work on my mood. At those times, I inevitably return to the work of Chester Pierce (Griffith 1998), the Harvard public health intellectual. He advanced the notion of extreme environments like prisons and submarines, comparing them, not surprisingly, to America's urban ghettos and their detrimental psychological effects. Environments can affect psychological healing processes.

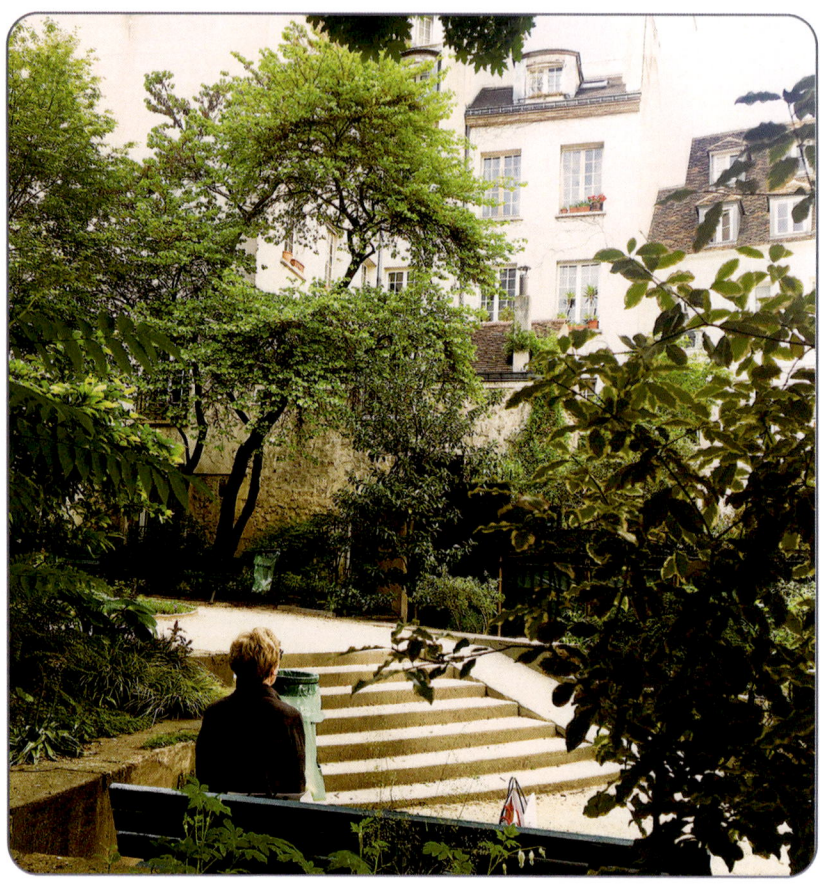

**Figure 6.1** Danielle-Mitterrand Garden, Paris, France.

This small well-kept public space, located on Rue de Bièvre, is known for its quiet isolation and attractive layout.

*Source.* Photograph by R. C. Grantham, AIA.

# Lingering in a Garden[2]

Shams al-Din Hafiz Shirazi asked, "What more has earth to give?" in a 14th-century poem called "To Linger in a Garden Fair." I wondered about the answer after a recent visit to Bournville, a residential

---

[2] Adapted with permission from Griffith EEH: Lingering in a Garden. *Psychiatric News*, September 2019. Copyright © 2019 American Psychiatric Association. All rights reserved.

*Focusing on Place*

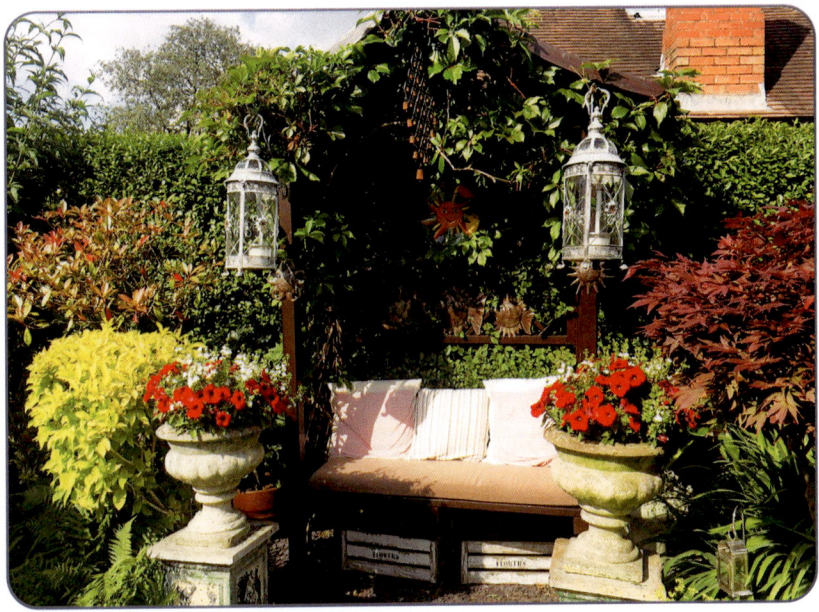

**Figure 6.2**  Open-Garden Day at Vinwood Garden in Birmingham, United Kingdom.

This unique garden surrounds a relatively modest home and offers seclusion for private discussions, reverie, and quiet examination of flora.

*Source.*   Photograph by Ezra E. H. Griffith, M.D.

neighborhood in the British city of Birmingham. I was invited to an open-garden day that the village residents attend each year. Bournville is considered Britain's original garden community (Figure 6.2). It eventually became a member of the U.K.'s National Garden Scheme. This organization encourages local neighborhoods to open their gardens to the public and charge entrance fees that are then donated to a charity. I chose my arrival at a garden called Vinwood to coincide with the half-hour entertainment of the Bournville Clarinet Choir. Its performance enhanced the entire afternoon's magical ambience. I lingered there for about 4 hours, conversing with other visitors and the property owners. The rich soft grass underfoot enticed the audience to sit and listen to the choir's performance of music by Dvorak.

The house was not imposingly large, and its lawns at the front, back, and one side were surrounded by 5-foot-high hedges. This made the lawns look like separate rooms, each with a different arrangement of intimate corners offering onlookers a chance to sit and peer through the underbrush. The plants and flowers at the edges of the lawns camouflaged a bench here; an armchair there; masks, mirrors, pots and pans reconfigured and repurposed; and small statues.

The owners of the property developed the garden partly as a sanctuary. They acknowledged that it required great manual effort but agreed that the work made time pass quickly and allowed them to relax as they admired the benefits of their labor. They enjoyed working together and supporting the plants' efforts to thrive. They were pleased to contribute to their community. At times, they entered the garden dispirited but always came out uplifted. Some visitors commented that the garden's beauty distracted them from their problems, and the flowers' perfumes were refreshing. The landscapes slowed them down and forced them to look around imaginatively. There was also the ineffable sensation of being held briefly captive in a space for meditation. As I watched the visitors strolling on the garden's narrow stone pathways, I couldn't help but smile. Everyone seemed entranced, putting names I didn't know to the plants and describing the flowers' colors with a knowledgeable vocabulary that was beyond mine.

We know that these relatively passive activities help people live longer. There are also benefits to sitting on a bench in a beautifully designed floral alcove chatting with friends and neighbors. The activity enhances social networking and reduces stress. That is why a colleague recently told me about the Biophilic Cities Network, which is committed to improving the connection between city residents and urban nature. After all, Vinwood is in a city but seems to bring the country into the urban space.

What more indeed does the earth have to give? Well, some answers have been discussed by Ephral Livni (2016) in a piece called "The Japanese Practice of 'Forest Bathing' Is Scientifically Proven to Improve Your Health." Just being in the presence of trees can have a positive effect on one's stress level and immune system.

## The House by the Sea[3]

The landscapes and seascapes caught by the camera in this 2017 film are enough to tempt anyone to sit and wait for the story to unfold. The villa sits high up overlooking the sea at the very water's edge, pointing

---

[3] Adapted with permission from Griffith EEH: The House by the Sea. *Psychiatric News*, September 2022. Copyright © 2022 American Psychiatric Association. All rights reserved.

*Focusing on Place*

me to the hypnotizing scenes I have seen in Croatia and, of course, in Barbados. However, this film is set in the South of France. It is named *La Villa* in French and marketed as *The House by the Sea* for Anglophone audiences. Written and directed by Robert Guédiguian and running for 107 minutes, the movie focuses on the transactions taking place within a finely crafted family space. The film was screened at the 74th Venice International Film Festival.

The movie opens with the camera riveted on the patriarch of the family. The action is slow. We understand eventually that he has had a cerebrovascular accident. We see him later in a wheelchair or a bed, presumably following his return home from hospital. He neither speaks nor moves. He has lost his ability to comprehend anything. He just stares ahead unflinchingly. It is around this impaired family elder that the story unfolds. His rigid body deflects the soliloquies that his offspring aim at him. The camera melds people and the stunning beauty of the region.

The major cast of characters is relatively small. Angèle is the daughter in her 60s who returns home to participate in the discussions about what now needs to be done. About what, you ask. Well, one might say that is the focus of the film. She is a successful actress, accustomed to all the drama on stage. However, she is not adept at dealing with difficult situations in her life. She left home a couple of decades ago, right after her young daughter drowned when left in the care of the patriarch. The girl's father never forgave Angèle for the accident, and he left town. Angèle nourished a grudge against her father. Her two losses kept her estranged from the villa and the patriarch for decades. Her pent-up rage, the shame, and the disgust found room just below the surface. So, when Benjamin, a young fisherman from the area who idolizes the famous actress, declares his interest in her, the defrosting of her protective guard takes a while. It comes partly because he can recite by heart snippets of Paul Claudel's writing and because he is persistent. Her face slowly loses its fixed glare. Benjamin takes her out in his fishing boat. The rippling waves wipe away years of tears and lamentations.

There are two brothers. One is the writer, Joseph, who returns for the family reunion accompanied by a fiancée half his age. Viewers will see him differently, perhaps as a failed hippie intellectual or as someone searching for Zion. He is evidently unhappy. The other sibling is Armand, who remained at home and runs the family restaurant. There is always disappointment in those who stay home, care for the first generation, and complain about not being appreciated by siblings who left. Armand is good friends with a couple who live next door. They have stayed home, too, and retired. But the going is financially rough for them. Of especial note is their unwillingness to accept help from their attentive and supportive physician-son who takes pleasure in offering money to lighten his parents' load. The parents eventually find peace in a collaborative suicide pact. The medic decides to leave the town after he has seduced Joseph's fiancée. They promise to connect in London.

There are others, disconnected from the villa, who occasionally enter the narrative. First come a trio of young illegal immigrants. Then there is a team of soldiers seeking the illegal migrants. Among them is a Black soldier who brings up the race question in every other sentence he addresses to people from whom he seeks information. These are irrelevancies in an otherwise tight storyline. One might still connect them to the main theme because of the uncertainty of the central characters' futures. There is change in the air because real estate agents and developers are snooping around.

Suddenly, the film becomes a wonderful stimulus for discussion, within a general or psychiatric educational context, of a circumscribed home-space. What is the patriarch's psychiatric and legal status? Does he need a guardian? Is the neighbors' decision to die by suicide justifiable? Do the three siblings need psychiatric or pastoral care? Might a psychiatrist be helpful in contributing to the development of a firmer family structure, undergirding maintenance of the villa and the restaurant? Should the siblings make new commitments to people and the place by the sea?

## C.L.R. James' *Beyond a Boundary*[4]

I was looking forward to attending the widely advertised C.L.R. James Distinguished Lecture to be delivered on the Barbados campus of the University of the West Indies by Professor Sir Hilary Beckles, vice-chancellor of the university. The occasion celebrated the 60th anniversary of the 1963 publication of *Beyond a Boundary* (reissued in 1993 and later by Duke University Press), which has become known as C.L.R. James' classic text on the history, sociology, and psychology of cricket. I have cited James liberally in my writing on leisure activities and their connection to the notions of belonging and therapeutic landscapes. I also featured him in my teaching about the scholarly contributions

---

[4] Adapted with permission from Griffith EEH: C.L.R. James' *Beyond a Boundary*. *Psychiatric News*, May 2023. Copyright © 2023 American Psychiatric Association. All rights reserved.

of Caribbean figures (such as Austin Clarke, Derek Walcott, George Lamming, and V. S. Naipaul) to the literature on social justice. It should be obvious then that the book is about much more than just cricket.

Cyril Lionel Robert James (1901–1989) is known as a Trinidadian historian, journalist, and Marxist who made a place for himself in the contested arena of colonial politics and public cultural criticism. He wrote on diverse subjects and in a variety of literary forms, often using a captivating prose. That night, I wanted to hear more about James and how he came to write a book about a sport while making astute observations about ethics, caste, and race matters in the colonial and postcolonial context of the Caribbean. Professor Beckles, the lecturer, is an established public critic and historian of cricket. He is also a potent voice for the reparations movement inside and outside the postindependence West Indies. Notable, too, is that he leads a university with a prestigious Faculty of Sport.

The lecture turned out to be a simultaneous commentary on sports and life. James's unique approach in his text was to look at colonial society from the Trinidadian angle, focusing on the intriguing sociopsychological space of cricket. The British had implanted this bat-and-ball game throughout its empire with varying success. As Sir Hilary stated in his presentation, there was little theater in the 20th-century British Caribbean, which therefore allowed cricket to fill that void. The playing field became the stage where the White colonizer lived out his dreams of dominance and superiority. James understood that it was also the place where the Black colonized could attend seriously to the master's edicts and improve on them. Cricket was ultimately not just leisure and amusement; it became a tool within the broader culture, linked to personal identity and dignity. The West Indies cricket team eventually found its place in international cricket circles with Blacks as team captains.

As I sat in the lecture hall, I recognized that James had framed cricket, the most prestigious sport in the British Caribbean (above even European football), within the complex culture of the British West Indies. James admitted that he was a good cricketer, but not one who had played at the international level. However, he could analyze the finer points of the game while pointing out that competitive sports was in many ways interconnected with the inequities and injustices of a colonized society. He justified his pronouncements in *Beyond a Boundary* with more than a modicum of arrogance. As he wrote "I did not merely play cricket. I studied it. I analysed strokes, I studied types, I read its history, its beginnings, how and when it changed from period to period, I read about it in Australia and in South Africa, I made clippings, I talked to all cricketers" (James 1963/1993, pp. 32–33).

He was as attentive to cricket as he was to literature and proud that he had pursued both. Noting that he had a profound liking for cricket and English literature, he concluded that his sense of conduct and morals came from these two preoccupations. He knew that the sociopolitical transformation that had to come in the broader colonized Caribbean society would be exemplified on the cricket pitch and reflected in the makeup of cricket teams. Sir Hilary hinted at all this in describing James's struggle with the publisher over the book's title: *Beyond a Boundary* or *Beyond the Boundary*.

Here is cricket as exemplar of the colonizer's structural classification in 1930s Trinidad cricket clubs. "The various first-class clubs represented the different social strata in the island within clearly defined bounds" (James 1963/1993, p. 49), he wrote. The Queen's Park Club was "top of the list" and "for the most part white and often wealthy" (James 1963/1993, p. 49). The second prestigious club was Shamrock, almost exclusively White and Catholic. Constabulary was made up of members of the local police force, all Black and captained by a White police inspector. There was Stingo, all Black and possessing no social status. James noted that for him, "Queen's Park and Shamrock were too high and Stingo was too low" (James 1963/1993, p. 50). There were two other clubs. One was "Maple, the club of the Brown-skinned middle class. Class did not matter so much to them as colour" (James 1963/1993, p. 50). The other club was "Shannon, the club of the black lower-middle class" (James 1963/1993, p. 50), with teachers and department store clerks, for example.

After much soul searching and seeking of advice from mentors, James joined Maple. He justified his decision by citing his achievements in the literary arts, while pointing courageously, I suggest, to his wish to keep company with individuals of a lighter complexion. He conceded that it was a costly decision full of social and political implications. Cricket had taught James the fundamental principles of loyalty to people, principles, and institutions. Racialized living was praxis, something more than the contours of theory.

## An Afternoon Constitutional[5]

It was a good day, one of those featuring a pleasant spring temperature and a sky that was boastfully blue. Since my destination was only about a mile away, I decided to take what my father used to call an

---

[5] Adapted with permission from Griffith EEH: An Afternoon Constitutional. *Psychiatric News*, June 2023. Copyright © 2023 American Psychiatric Association. All rights reserved.

afternoon constitutional (defined in his 30-year-old *American Heritage Dictionary* as a walk taken for one's health) and daydream on the way. Young undergraduates moved swiftly around me, engaged in their own pressing business. When I turned a corner to reach the Yale Beinecke Rare Book and Manuscript Library, there were more students seated casually at occasional tables, deep into their computers and ignoring passersby. The peace and quiet made the daffodils and tulips stand out. Everybody seemed to appreciate the privilege of enjoying lethargy and calm. I had two thoughts. I wondered about the money and effort taken to create and maintain a campus space so conducive to feeling at ease. Then I recognized the contrast with the reports and debates on daily television.

The Beinecke Library houses a large collection dedicated to rare books and manuscripts and serves as a repository of literary archives. Examples of its holdings are the Gutenberg Bible that dates to 1454 and a 1,250-year-old print of Buddhist prayers from Japan. The library was opened in October 1963 and has steadily become a special place within the university. This is not just because of its holdings, the exquisite courtyard, and its outstanding architecture (like its 1.25-inch thick "windows" made of translucent Vermont marble panels that protect the collections from sunlight). The library has earned a reputation for its programs of concerts, readings, and conferences that are diverse and attract students, faculty, and the public. It is easy to see how the Beinecke defines and extends the mission of a university, promoting community unity and quietly enhancing mutual pursuit of intellectual curiosity.

I had set out from home on that recent afternoon to be in the audience at the Beinecke for the Yale Collegium Musicum's performance of music from Renaissance Italy (Figure 6.3). Another look into my father's dictionary informed me that *collegium* refers to "a group, the members of which pursue shared goals while working within a framework of mutual trust and respect." The Yale Collegium, featuring both singers and instrumentalists, reportedly gave its first concert in 1943. Its mission was apparently defined as the performance of music from the 12th through the 18th centuries. Not being an aficionado of Italian Renaissance music, I think I was drawn to the concert because of the performance venue and my love of singing. The event also represented a cultural happening, open to the community and free of charge.

A preconcert presentation and Rebecca Arkenberg's (2002) article "Music in the Renaissance" (posted on The Metropolitan Museum of Art's website) pointed out that Italian Renaissance music was played

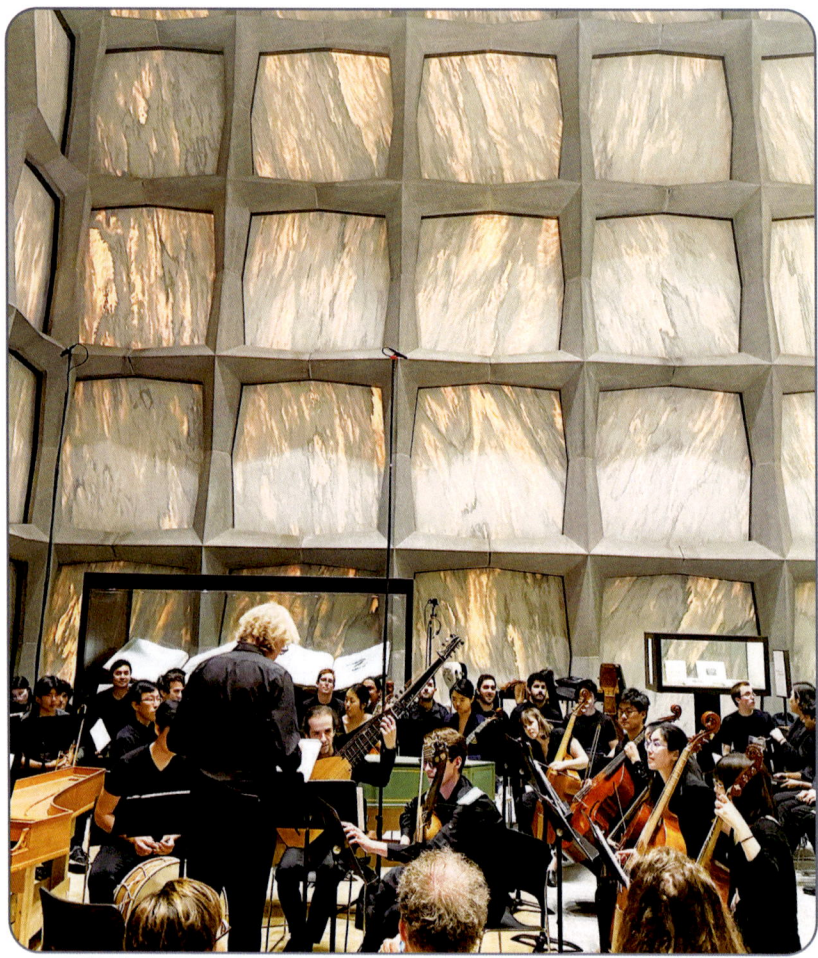

**Figure 6.3** Italian Renaissance Music in New Haven, Connecticut.

The Yale Collegium Musicum performs music from Renaissance Italy at a public concert in Yale's Beinecke Rare Book and Manuscript Library.

*Source.* Photograph by Brigitte Griffith.

in the 15th and 16th centuries. Polyphony, the singing of multiple lines of music at the same time, had become fashionable. Two major forms of polyphony developed. Motets were composed using texts from religious sources, and the madrigal employed excerpts from secular sources like poems.

The concert I attended began with a "lauda," described in the program as a devotional song composed "to be sung by lay people outside of the official liturgy of the Catholic mass." There was also a four-part madrigal composed by Philippe Verdolot, one of the famous composers of the genre. That piece was in sharp contrast to the "lamentation" (a plaintive composition for a single voice) composed by Claudio Monteverdi. That obviously mournful work was based on a text, "So sweet is the torment that resides in my breast, that I live content … at the gates of heaven." "The Triumph of Love," composed by Giaches de Vert, another madrigal expert, was performed before the program transitioned to popular tunes, which, to my ear, sounded more rhythmic and danceable.

About 50 singers and instrumentalists performed with sensitivity and a structured delicacy. The music felt familiar to me, I suspect, because of contact with English composers like William Byrd and the chorales of the period from other parts of Europe. This genre of experience never fails to make me contemplate my own pathway to a university life. I knew instinctively that I could not have attended a concert like this one in 1950s Barbados, especially in a building of such intentional magnificence. I enjoyed thinking back to the instruments I encountered in my childhood: the occasional violin, the guitar for folk music, and the ubiquitous church organ. Then, once I migrated to the United States, I met an Italian youngster who played classical guitar. At this Beinecke concert, I was introduced to the theorbo, dulcian, and sackbut. What a revelation!

I could not help moving from this performance of Italian Renaissance music in a beautiful university space to the persistent contentious noise about equitable access to these distinguished precincts. Watching the young people singing this music and playing these instruments with such passion and vigor was, to use their own patois, awesome. They could see the breadth of what was possible for them in their universe. The obligation, then, must be to reinforce the commitment to equitable access for youths to these spaces.

## Archiving Our Pasts[6]

Old photographs and other memorabilia have a special importance for many of us. Saving them helps us keep our family members interconnected. In my case, I have long held tightly to my father's gift of

---

[6] Adapted with permission from Griffith EEH: Archiving Our Pasts. *Psychiatric News*, July 2023. Copyright © 2023 American Psychiatric Association. All rights reserved.

his 1936 edition of the two-volume *Webster's Universal Dictionary* and the undated edition of Robert Young's *Analytical Concordance to the Bible*. These objects are not yet ready for distribution! Processing these notions of archiving, I immediately remembered a friend who recently donated a collection of stuffed animals to someone with a young child. There were two puppets in the collection, I was told, which the donor had used to communicate with a younger sister. She was hoping the beneficiaries of the gift would reproduce this wonderful experience within their own family.

A woman who migrated years ago from France to the United States carefully kept pictures and documents that reflect details of her life-long history. The picture and marriage certificate (Figures 6.4 and 6.5) come from her family archive and focus on the 1911 wedding of her maternal grandparents. The photograph was taken in the department of Moselle, a region in northeast France. This geographic area had been under German occupation since the 1870s, which accounts for the German language used in the official document. The region reverted to France at the end of the First World War and experienced similar upheaval between 1939 and 1945. The archive's owner pointed out the details of the figures in the picture: their stylized clothing and coiffures, the top hat and white gloves, and their personal bearing. The photograph is an important reference point, as she got to know these relatives only from about the late 1950s.

The Oakland Museum of California recently hosted an exhibition about Angela Yvonne Davis, the feminist and avowed Communist so beloved by the political left. She is a prolific scholar concerned with matters of class, gender, race, and prison affairs. It turned out that some of the material displayed in the museum program came from the collection of the community archivist Lisbet Tellefsen. On show was, for example, a stunning group of posters pulled together over the years that featured the visage of Angela Davis. In conjunction with the exposition, Tellefsen and two other archivists, Damien McDuffie and Odette Pollar, staged a didactic presentation about community archiving. The program title, "Preserving Black Memory: A Conversation With Oakland Culture Keepers," captured their interest in safeguarding memories about the Black community and reinforcing citizens' identities and personal pride.

These unique audiovisual lectures and conversations held the audience's interest and provoked considerable interchange during the question-and-answer period. The speakers described their collecting as a strategy for keeping Black history alive. However, I also saw their

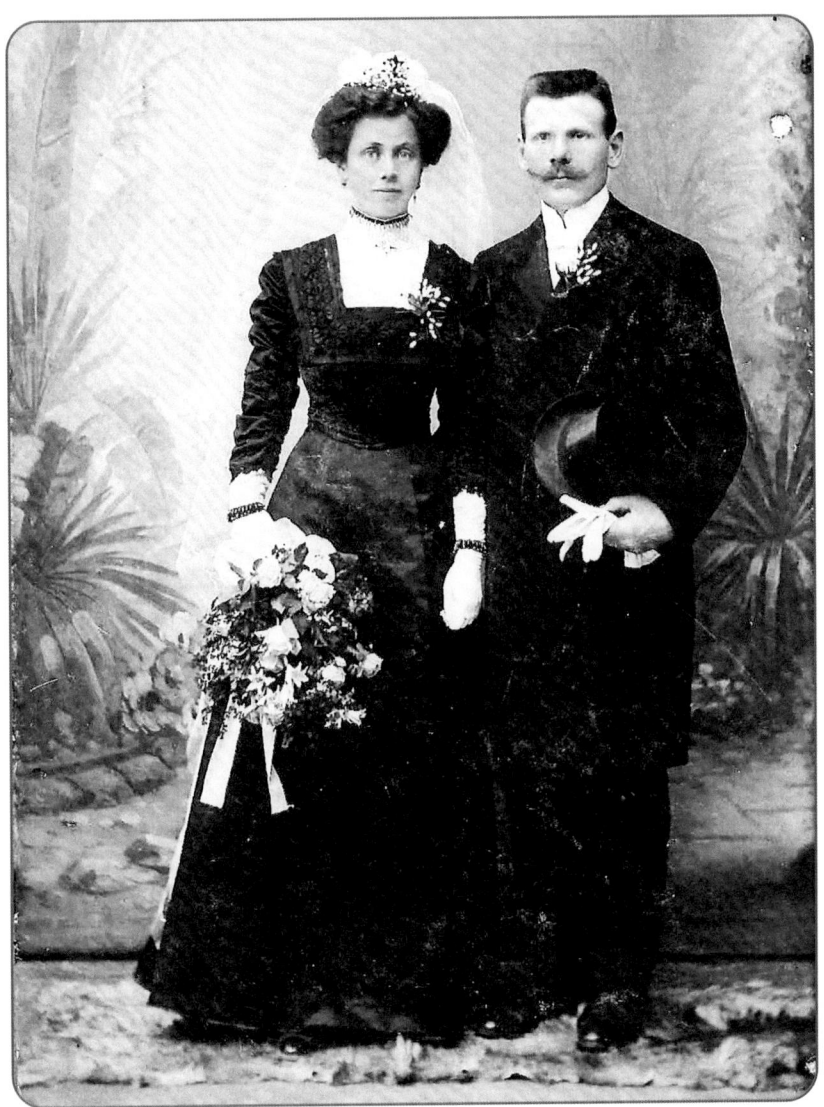

**Figure 6.4** Private Family Archiving.

A 1911 photograph of the wedding of a French émigré's grandparents. This is just one of the documents that the woman carefully kept that archive her life-long history in considerable detail.

*Source.* Private Anonymous Collection. Used with permission. Photograph credit: Brigitte Griffith.

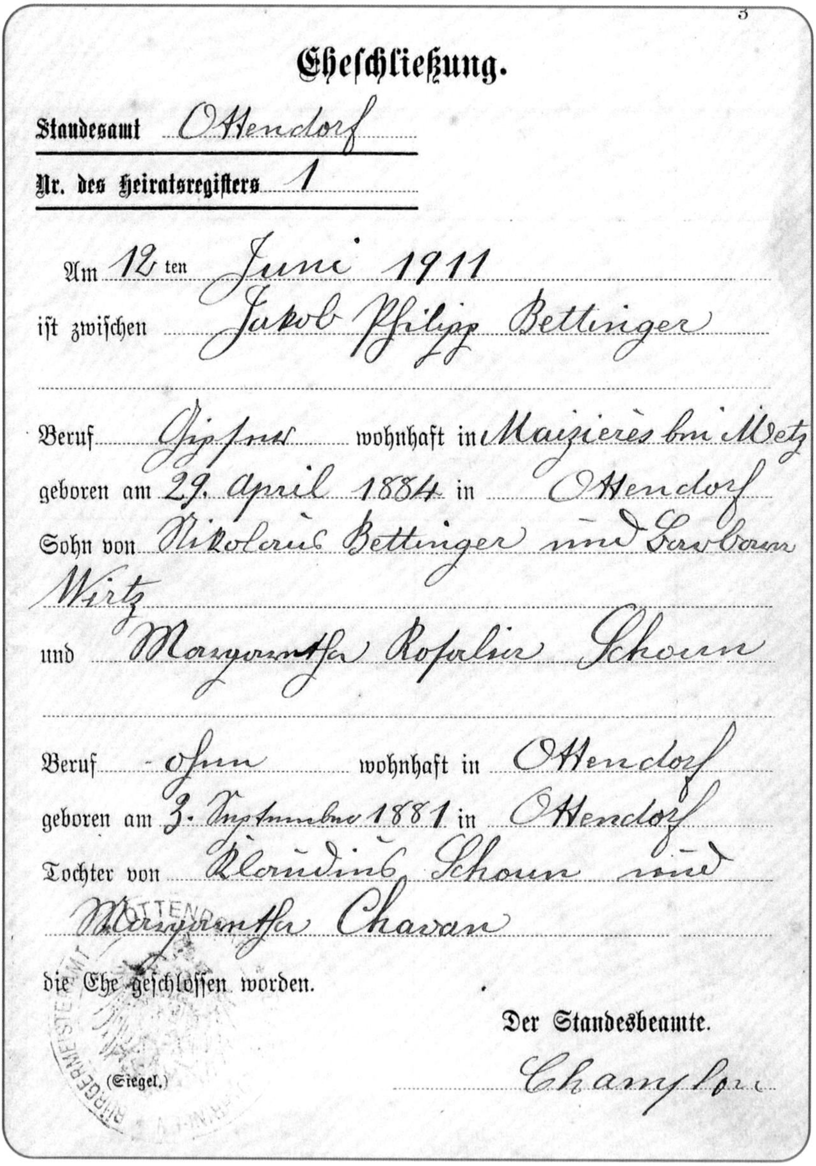
3

Eheschließung.

Standesamt Ottendorf

Nr. des Heiratsregisters 1

Am 12ten Juni 1911

ist zwischen Jakob Philipp Bettinger

Beruf Gipser wohnhaft in Maizières bei Metz

geboren am 29. April 1884 in Ottendorf

Sohn von Nikolaus Bettinger und Barbara Wirtz

und Margaretha Rosalie Schoun

Beruf ohne wohnhaft in Ottendorf

geboren am 3. September 1881 in Ottendorf

Tochter von Claudius Schoun und Margaretha Chavan

die Ehe geschlossen worden.

Der Standesbeamte.

(Siegel.) Champlon

**Figure 6.5** Private Family Archiving.

A 1911 photograph of the marriage certificate of a French émigré's grandparents. This is just one of the documents that the woman carefully kept that archive her lifelong history in considerable detail.

*Source.* Private Anonymous Collection. Used with permission. Photograph credit: Brigitte Griffith.

efforts as having broad application to many cultures. Many people I know depend on safeguarding objects, information, principles, and rituals for future use. The presenters pointed to their involvement in childhood practices such as accumulating matchbooks and photographs. They also were exposed to relatives who had developed habits of putting aside groups of objects.

Tellefsen declared a penchant for materials with a political history. Hence, her interest in Angela Davis posters and other information about the Black Panther Party. Pollar demonstrated her attachment to a community club called "The Rainbow Sign." That organization facilitated gatherings of Blacks for social, political, and educational purposes. They held dance classes and poetry readings, for example, as Blacks had little access to this kind of community institution. McDuffie described his compulsion to take photographs of life in the Black community of Oakland, California. As the three lecturers talked, it became clearer how each had envisioned a way to put a personal imprint on some aspect of the local Black culture. They discussed several definitions of community archiving: keeping family history alive, preserving memories of a single institution, collecting materials that will provide information for future users, and engaging in activity that flows from visualizing oneself as part of history. The discussants encouraged members of the audience to engage in archival collecting, even while making clear that preserving and passing on collections to others remain complicated tasks.

Returning to the French family archive, the picture and document provide some insight into the hardships that flowed from the cultural, linguistic, and political changes forced by several major wars. This archivist recalled having to speak German with some relatives who spoke no French. She also noted that individuals from this northeast area of France, who had been raised in this Franco-Germanic context, were stigmatized because they manipulated French with difficulty and spoke it with a German accent. They seemed out of step with the aesthetics of French life. In private, they talked of feeling like outsiders.

The archive's owner takes pride in a family line that stretches historically over 100 years or so. She understands the subtleties of caste and culture and bristles at the oversimplification of discrimination and othering. She argues passionately that information about one's origins helps us all withstand the arrogant claims of those who advocate maintenance of the caste ladder because they like being on its dominant rungs. The archived past gives clarity to one's present vision of things.

## On Radishes and Other Culinary Memories[7]

I have had the good fortune to open the door of my home, after returning from a competitive soccer match, to be engulfed by an enticing aroma coming from the oven. The baker had been at work. It all compensated for my losing the game. On other occasions, I have been served a mixture of *reine claude* plums and apricots and heard the fruit whispering, "Someone cares about you." Food has a place among tales of people, places, and health. Memories of cuisine reassure me about the rhythms of mundane life. They tell me that things are all right, in good order. Friends have similar reactions about music or art in their lives. So, I have become bolder in the recounting of cuisine stories linked to sights and smells and events. Food marks lived experiences of kindness, joy, and companionship and, from time to time, also of disappointment and irritability.

There is a favorite fish restaurant where I go to celebrate special events. Its introductory offering (the *amuse-bouche*) is frequently a plate of pink radishes for the table, accompanied by salt, butter, and a basket of bread. Every time I attend a meal in that restaurant, I go through the same ritual: I ask someone nearby why people like to eat radishes. The answer includes mention of the vegetable's spicy, crunchy taste, which is enhanced by butter and salt. There is, too, its contributions to good health: anticancer effects, addition of vitamin C to the diet, minimal calorie load, and fiber and roughage for the digestive system. The explanation evaporates quickly. Then I settle in to revisit the memory that always leaves me thankful.

I have no recollection, as a young Barbadian, of ever eating a radish. It is about 50 years since I first encountered that pink root vegetable on a visit to a French family. The parents of a medical student friend had invited me to spend the weekend at their home. The mother was very solicitous, clearly wishing me to be comfortable and relaxed. She tried hard to make sure her kitchen served hospitality and kindness. The pink radishes were a surprise. I did not even know how to proceed, and I had to watch everyone at the table to see what they would do. The mother noticed my disarray. I knew I was not smiling.

As the first radish entered my mouth, I felt the tingling and slightly bitter taste spread over my tongue and the involuntary grimace take

---

[7] Adapted with permission from Griffith EEH: On Radishes and Other Culinary Memories. *Psychiatric News*, September 2023. Copyright © 2023 American Psychiatric Association. All rights reserved.

over my face. It would have been perceived even by a blind person. There was no point trying to utter something about liking it. My hostess did not miss a beat. She reassured me that she had planned for such a contretemps. Something else was available. She was an endearing mother who recognized that I was far from home and missing family and friends. She invited me at other occasions, always making sure I learned something new about French culture while she engaged patiently and with elegance her curiosity about Barbados. She passed on years ago, but her physician son is still a good friend. We have talked often about cultural differences and adaptation.

Another story, this time about Black Forest cake, is worth the telling. I was offered a slice as dessert while visiting a small village in the Lorraine region of France. I was among friends sometime in the 1970s, enjoying the camaraderie. Someone explained that this gateau was a specialty of a nearby patisserie (now closed, I have learned). On first view, the red cherries, placed on cream with chocolate shavings, made an enticing tableau. Closer examination revealed the layers of chocolate cake sandwiched between more cream and cherries. I gradually discovered the kirsch that slightly dented the sweetness of the fruit. I have tasted many different versions of Black Forest cake since then, but all have fallen short of that first contact with perfection. A few days ago, I tried a piece from a cake in which the chef had replaced the chocolate cake with chocolate mousse. Well done, I agreed, but not reaching the original yet. In any event, there was no accompanying laughter, banter, or youthful gaiety in the air. The original tasting cemented the feeling of friendship, support, and mutual respect.

The final story is about oxtails, a special Barbados dish that I recall now because one of its expert creators recently lost his wife. She was a close relative. He set the rules and standards of how to eat oxtails, which is with the pads of your fingers. The thumb is placed on one edge of vertebra bone and the forefinger on the other edge. The cylinder of meat and bone is then delicately brought to the mouth. It is a societal transgression to eat oxtails with cutlery. Perfection of the grasp is essential, as it is a firm hold that facilitates sucking of the bone. Food enthusiasts will try to compare this sacred act to eating roasted bone marrow. That is a wasteful effort, as roasted bone marrow does not offer the pleasure of oxtail meat and culinary spices that include some type of pepper sauce. Similarly, serving oxtail meat off the bone is pointless creativity, as there is no bone to enjoy. Still, the practice may be found among the uninitiated in the art of oxtail adoration. Barbadian sucking of oxtail bones with meat and condiments memorializes the joy of communal eating. It reinforces a sense of belonging to a group and defines family. Appreciating this underscores the final prohibition: the one against eating oxtails in solitude. If there is no other option, well, fine. On the other hand, any psychiatrist who understands food will ask why one would want to eat oxtails by oneself. Think about it. Alone? By the way, you must have napkins available.

## Photography as a Mirror With Memory[8]

I recently attended the 2023 James Weldon Johnson Memorial Lecture given by the poet Robin Coste Lewis on the Yale campus. She delivered an address that partly involved simultaneously reading poetry and presenting photographs that came from her grandmother's collection. She was melding poetry (a form of narrative) and photography. As the talk unfolded, my thoughts returned periodically to an exhibition I visited at the Pompidou Center in Paris, France, only a few weeks ago called "Corps à Corps: Histoire(s) de la Photographie" ("Body to Body: History(ies) of Photography"). I was reminded that for the last decade or so, I have witnessed the increasing influence of photography on different forms of narrative.

The Paris exposition presented two collections of photography, one public from the National Museum of Modern Art and the other private from the filmmaker Marin Karmitz. The photographs dated from early 20th century to contemporary works and focused on human beings and narratives. The curators devised a seven-part classification system that gave the exhibition structure and made it easier to follow commentary in the program notes. They enunciated principles for exploration of this type of artistic venture and framed several questions for consideration: Is it important to keep an eye on the relationship between photographer and subject? Is that connection defined by power, complicity, or rejection? Is photography principally a medium of introspection, or may we see it also as a mirror with a memory? And finally, besides the photographer, does the audience have some responsibility for the photographed subjects?

I tried to make sense of the Robin Lewis lecture and to establish a connection between her work and the structural principles that I had

---

[8] Adapted with permission from Griffith EEH: Photography as a Mirror With Memory. *Psychiatric News*, December 2023. Copyright © 2023 American Psychiatric Association. All rights reserved.

gleaned from the Paris exhibition. I could only do so readily by keeping in mind how I had employed photography in my own scholarship. I had in fact done so in two ways: in a study of leadership and membership in a Barbados Indigenous religious group and in thinking about Black autobiographies. In the first instance, photography was essential in illustrating what Paris curators would call the "interiors" of my religious study group, which is to say, "a place apart, governed by rules, modes of operation and temporalities entirely of its own." The curators even recalled Michel Foucault's original term "heterotopy" as they explained how one can find freedom as well as isolation in these spaces. In the second instance of biographical use, I was more likely to focus on images of faces or places. So, in my reflections, I felt I was making some connection to the structure offered by the Paris exhibition and was also appreciating Lewis's integration of poetry and photography.

In the group of photographs labeled *The First Faces* (*Visages*) from the Paris exhibit, the curators pointed out that it could be taken for granted that in the act of photography, exploration of the human body starts with the face. Such images represent the first step toward a relationship between photographer and subject. Anonymous faces, without social context, could well be the pretext for further study of the face. Photography of one's visage is an act of engagement and renders the subject visible. Viewers encountering the image may have a pleasant experience while formulating questions about the subject's identity. Examples of the relationship between these theoretical notions and the photographs used to illustrate this category were pictures of the European Gypsy community in the 1950s and of children forced to work in American factories during the early 20th century.

The curators discussed another group labeled *Within Oneself* (*En Soi*). Pictures in this group showed individuals seemingly absorbed in their own thoughts. The photographer seems detached from the goings-on being recorded. Alternatively, the photographer may present the image with considerable empathy. The curators noted that some artists may rely on technical ability with the camera, utilizing light and shadow to create certain moods like solitude or sadness. They also referenced images of bodies in trance, which made me think of church members, from my research projects, dancing while possessed by the Holy Spirit.

I enjoyed perusing another category of photographs labeled *Flashes* (*Fulgurances*). The notes described this as photography occurring in a moment. "The photographer stands and waits for the image to appear." There is a capturing of the micro-period and a sort of grasping of the other. It may also be a way to reveal relationships between human

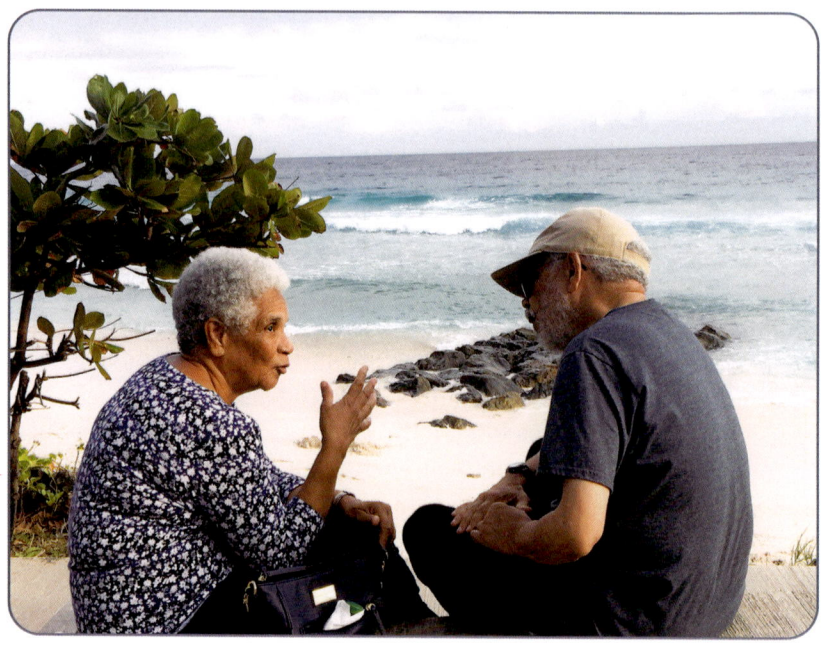

**Figure 6.6** A Brother and Sister Talk.

This photograph captures a private conversation between two siblings in a public park, Barbados.

*Source.* Private Anonymous Collection. Used with permission. Photograph credit: Brigitte Griffith.

beings. Examples of this form were pictures taken on the street, of someone on a subway, and of a couple dancing. I found this to be also a potentially intrusive category. Flashes were a common form of photography during the early years of the civil rights movement, with snapshots of ubiquitous racialized incidents illustrating hatred and fear and incidents of White privilege gone mad.

I close this column with a 2017 photograph, *A Brother and Sister Talk* (Figure 6.6), that captured me in private conversation with my sister. The photograph reflected the interaction, the proximity of bodies, the uncrowded Barbadian beach, the blessing of familial nearness, and the religion-tinged tranquility. We, the subjects, were unaware of any camera. As devout a Christian as my sister was, our conversations always ended on promise and assurance. No formal leave-taking—just a mutual and traditional Bajan "I gone." As that beautiful hymn, the one that she sometimes sang as a contralto soloist, states, she was confident that if the Almighty's eye was on the sparrow, He was also watching her. That photograph's moment I guard jealously.

# Dreaming With Freud[9]

There are three criteria that promise me a wonderful evening of play-watching at small Paris theaters: a production that lasts around 75 minutes, uses one or two actors, and features superb artists with established reputations. These three standards were easily met in *Freud et la Femme de Chambre* (*Freud and the Housekeeper*). The play, written by Leonardo de la Fuente, was directed by Alain Sachs and put on at the Montparnasse Theater. Nassima Benchicou as Marie and François Berléand as Sigmund Freud were featured in a splendid production. It turned out to be full of witty interchange between the duo of actors while also evoking serious contemplation of Freud's work. This was not at all a highbrow approach to the master's contributions. It was more of a hilarious, comical drama that involved popular concepts like the unconscious and applications of dream theory and psychoanalysis.

The setting was a large hotel room in 1923 Rome, Italy, and the entire play unfolded in that circumscribed space. There was an ensuite bathroom whose door opened and closed on occasion, giving depth to the room. We never see its interior. However, it served as a prop for some very amusing banter full of hints and speculation, none of which led to any overt sexual contact. Sigmund Freud never gives in to temptation, no matter from which angle it approached. There was a large window on one side of the room that permitted the housekeeper to interact with people passing in the street below. We could hear neighborhood activity, as when military troops or Marie's friends passed by. Italy was in political turmoil at the time, but the play only hints at that connection. In fact, we learn nothing about the reason for Freud's visit to Rome with his daughter Anna.

There was a large bed with its head against the room's main wall, on which hangs a crucifix. The bed is a curious center of attention, as much provocative action and verbal exchange take place on and around it. I laugh as I note that Marie the housekeeper will jump on and off it, sit on it, and stretch out on it for analysis. She will do as she very well wishes, but that bed will be used only for talk and sleep.

---

[9] Adapted with permission from Griffith EEH: Dreaming With Freud. *Psychiatric News*, June 2024. Copyright © 2024 American Psychiatric Association. All rights reserved.

And the audience will laugh at the outrageousness of it all. Sexuality was in the air, but never concretized. Sometimes a bed is just, well, for sleeping. This, mind you, is in the context where Marie is outfitted in a housekeeper's uniform that enhances her very attractive figure, giving her space to romp and strike a variety of poses, without more, as the lawyers say.

At the play's debut, Freud is in his bed asleep. Marie knocks, and since there is no answer, she enters and proceeds to open the blinds that will surely cause him to wake up. He is upset by the disturbance. However, the conversation starts with his inquiry about who she is, while she feigns ignorance about him. We quickly find out that she had met him when she was 10 years old and hoped for another encounter to cultivate a relationship. She had even dreamt about him, which piques his curiosity. She also reveals she thought that he was a circus hypnotist, a theatrical shot that is delivered almost imperceptibly. He insists he uses hypnotism to heal people.

The play proceeds with skillful directorial guidance, and Marie is soon posing the questions—not with analytic precision, but with guileless insouciance. The dialogue goes in several directions, with deeper and deeper probing on both sides. The play's author and director illustrate playfully Freud's mannerisms. At one point, he is lying on the bed, and Marie is sitting in a chair slowly stroking her chin. Another time, she replies to him with flair and condescension, "Je comprends" (I understand), and the audience rolls in laughter at the impeccable timing. Freud gradually cedes territory. We learn some important information.

He tells her about a dream and gives her his interpretation of it. At the center of his formulation is his father. Marie uses her own down-to-earth approach and concludes that the dream is about Freud himself. She has no skills to debate and closes the matter with the suggestion that her conclusion speaks for itself. She seems to have a point. After all, he was talking as though his logic was flawless, while she framed her reasoning in a plain, intuitive way, as her culture would have dictated. He also noted that there was a bubbly, upbeat spontaneity about her and her problem-solving that led him at one point to moan about his inability to find solutions to his own problems. He confessed that he was unable to define love or loss. The loss focused on the deaths of a daughter and a grandchild. Nothing else was said about love.

Other themes emerged in after-theater discussion with friends. One was Freud's denial of God's existence. It highlighted even more sharply his extensive mention of pain—concerning death and the ache he carried in his jaw that had required surgery. Put together, his complaints had surely contributed to the despondency that he described. I could not help feeling some sympathy for his emotional state, which was expressed so realistically by the actor. One could see some humility in his need for solace. He admitted his suffering and recognized somewhat that self-analysis was not effective succor. There was a scene toward the end where noise caused Marie to rush toward the window. Someone was hurt in the street below the hotel room. Marie turned and screamed at Freud to get help. He froze. She accused him of selfishness and wondered how he could be so self-absorbed and taken by his intellectual brooding and preoccupation with observation and analysis. She asked him about his apparent lack of interest in executing action to help others. In an incredible surprise, it turned out that the entire narrative was only a dream. Still, one is left with the practical question of how to meld active care with theorizing. And there is the frightening thought that, being human, we all have frailties and vulnerabilities that will, at some time, bring us low and dependent on others.

## Aging and Political Theater[10]

People from all walks of life were participating in the recent debate about candidates for political office and how they were aging. With all this talk, I still found it difficult to follow the lines of argument. One could readily find arrogance, bombast, and even denial in them. Some journalists insisted that one politician seemed stronger and more dynamic than another. Others felt they could look at a politician's gait and deduce whether he had the ability to carry out his duties. Observers demanded to see the medical records of the politicians they disliked. They believed they could make solid predictions about a specific person's future performance from yesterday's mental status examinations.

I wanted to put some structure back into my thinking. Luckily, I came across a recent biographical story by French journalist Charlotte Herzog (2024) called "Raconte-moi ta vieillesse" ("Tell me about your old age"), and I thought it worth sharing. Herzog begins by reminding us of a quote from Simone de Beauvoir: "La vieillesse, c'est ce qui arrive aux gens qui deviennent vieux" ("Old age is what happens to people

---

[10] Adapted with permission from Griffith EEH: Aging and Political Theater. *Psychiatric News*, September 2024. Copyright © 2024 American Psychiatric Association. All rights reserved.

who get old"). That statement reestablishes a sense of orderliness, even while it is full of circularity. Not many politicians easily admit to growing older. Could it be true that they gain experience while remaining young? Are they that different from us?

Herzog then introduces the reader to Nicole, an 84-year-old divorcée who spends every day in the same café in the Belleville section of Paris, sitting in the same seat at the same table from two to seven o'clock. Nicole has short, white hair, complains of sciatica in her left leg, and is surrounded by a pile of newspapers, a glass of water, and an espresso diluted by a bit of water, which the French call "un café allongé." She does not sleep well these days. She has a new printer that is complicated, and she is unable to handle certain maneuvers on her computer. She is worried that she may have to pay her taxes online this year.

From time to time sitting at her table, Nicole feels cold. She recognizes that her troublesome old person's chill starts from the inside and does not respond to the warmth offered by sweaters. But every day, she leaves her residence for the café, in part to avoid suddenly dying alone at home. That is what happened to her mother. Nicole admits to detesting all types of emptiness. She had a twin sister who died about 20 years ago in a train accident. Memories no longer come to her easily, and the days are not always pleasant. Sometimes she has arthritic pains, accompanied by anxiety and a touch of vertigo as she anticipates tomorrow's arrival.

She runs through her list of life events for Herzog: three children, an abortion, separations, a depressive episode at retirement, broken connections with two daughters, and grandchildren she knows only through photographs. She is familiar with physical solitude, as well as the isolation that is so difficult to put into words. She tells Herzog: "Les gens viennent et s'en vont" ("People come and they leave").

Enough about Nicole! However, I still want you to keep in mind the literary tableau of pathos and humility that Charlotte Herzog evokes: the memory lapses, the arthritis and sciatica, the secret fears of this and that, the search to retain dignity, and the loneliness and reconsideration of a past life. Not every old person's story goes down this path. Nevertheless, I found it a good exemplar of growing old.

What a contrast with the narratives of aging offered by the individuals seeking high political office in the United States. Some of them tend to avoid discussing the subject, even as they confront life anchored by the age-80 mark. They want to control the pace and direction of the aging process, which may include intellectual deterioration.

Their advisers tell anyone who will listen that if their candidate can effectively handle a specific cognitive task in the present, it is evidence that they can execute other functions as well. That is wishful thinking.

There is an amusing clamor, by fierce television critics, for testing opponents who are, say, near age 80. Younger candidates, still in their 70s, escape these demands, especially if they can talk confidently about their good health. This bluffing style is disarming and convinces the naïve that good health today necessarily means good health tomorrow. Those who espouse this view have never heard the Barbadian dialogue between two men chatting on a street corner. One says: "Boy, here today, gone tomorrow." The other replies, "No, man, it is here today and gone today."

The two men are reflecting on the uncertainty of life, which should temper arrogance in talking about aging. However, we cannot say about a particular person that the process will proceed in a certain way, with stops here and there for reflection and time to say goodbye to friends and enemies. Neither do we know the day and time when the end will come. But when we pursue political objectives, we find it easy to distort stories of aging to reach our desired goals.

Nicole's life story naturally seems chaotic and unpredictable, partly because of her minimal resources and pronounced isolation. Nevertheless, we should not be fooled by status, access to wealth, or the presence of witnesses and social support. Father Time eventually has his way when he is ready, despite the candidates' insistence on overseeing their lives. Their claims are mere political theater enjoyed by demanding audiences.

## Comments and Clinical Observations

I have often thought of Fiona Smyth's article (2005) on medical geography and therapeutic places as a landmark explanatory piece about the relationship between health and place. Smyth's work clarified for me how certain structured settings and situations might support or inhibit the unfolding of therapeutic processes. Smyth (2005), building on earlier scholarship such as that of W. M. Gesler (1992) in this arena, proposed three structural models. The first stated that certain environments, such as Lourdes in France, managed to develop and maintain a cultural reputation for healing. In Barbados, there is a specific spot along the island's western coast where for years a factory has discharged hot water into the sea just off the beach. Residents love to swim in that warm water, and they have christened the area "the pot," while celebrating its healing properties. Many people believe that the warm water alleviates arthritic pain and other ailments. In the second model, health care was manifest in the daily practices and rituals of institutions designated for that purpose, such as hospitals and clinics. The third model encompassed therapeutic networks specially arranged for support and care, such as groups organized in homes or places of worship. I remind readers that in Chapter 5, I discuss the multiple and varied functions of faith communities, including their role as healing communities.

In an earlier text (Griffith 2018), I discussed how the linking of health and place had expanded to include an unexpected assortment of spaces, such as gardens, homes, retreat centers, and even walking groups (Liamputtong and Suwankhong 2015). With this change, managers focused on the internal and external structures of these spaces, as well as the therapeutic or nontherapeutic nature of events occurring within them. I was intrigued by how loci, such as home-spaces and workspaces, might serve a therapeutic mission and ultimately perpetuate and disseminate this connection between health (including well-being) and place. I encourage clinicians to take a special interest in how place-space-geography may be used in their work. The concept adds a different dimension to thinking about the development and unfolding of an individual life. The notion of place adds depth, clarity, and specificity to the traditional, longitudinal, and time-based structure of adult development. In many cases, thinking about the space someone occupies permits a sharply defined, more granular examination of what an individual is doing with life.

Thus, in the interim between the appearance of Smyth's article and the present time, the development of the health-place link has blossomed. Colleagues in other disciplines are also bearing witness to the utility of the concept. For example, earlier in this chapter I mention an exhibition, titled "Personal Geographies," at the Yale Center for British Art. The focus is on the British painter Eileen Hogan, who maintains a special interest in portraits and landscapes. I leave it to the viewer to determine the quality of the interaction between these two fundamental elements. Conveying measured relaxation and a modicum of task-oriented activity, the exhibition illustrates the therapeutic aspects of limited work and active leisure.

I have already commented on the results that can be gleaned from systematic observations of goings-on within unique circumscribed spaces. Another column in this chapter, "The House by the Sea," represents distinctive creative efforts in the domain of cinema. The focus is on family members gathered in the home-space to contemplate the future care of the family patriarch. He has suffered a severe stroke and remains unable to care for himself. This is not a home caring for children. The needs are at the other end of the life cycle, and the adults all have competing needs and desires. The boundaries around the village facilitate a biopsychosocial examination of the goings-on. Place and health are inextricably intertwined.

The column about aging ("Aging and Political Theater") addresses, too, the final years of an individual's life. With advancing age, the spaces that Nicole, the column's subject, occupies are restricted. She can be found at home in the night and morning; in the afternoon and early evening, she sits in the same seat at the same table in the same neighborhood bistro. The familiarity of the two principal spaces that define her, with the camaraderie of individuals around her, help her contend with the solitude and boredom that mark her existence. The sharpened perimeter surrounding her daily space forces a clinician or narrator of her story to pose questions about her solitude, foreclosed interpersonal interactions with others, and views of personal contentment.

"Dreaming With Freud" was a remarkable exemplar of creativity, with the stage set in a European hotel room in the early part of the 20th century. Everything revolved around the psychoanalyst Freud. The bed at the center of the architecture was there for dreaming. The audience eventually recognized that the confined space was required to facilitate concentration on the action that carried double meanings with every utterance. In addition, the fascinating reality was that Freud is shown as a lonely sufferer, using the mechanism of dreaming to confront the occasional unhappiness of life. The theatrical use of a hotel bedroom to explore life's unpleasantness takes us away from the displeasure of encountering pain in our mundane spaces. The theater as landscape gives us room to look at the event and its secondary transactions from different angles. It may even be enjoyable to discuss the production over a meal with friends. This is a potent example of circumscribed spaces being used to focus on stories of human beings and their meaning.

Years ago, I delivered a short lecture to high school students at the reopening of their library. I spoke about the potential uses of such a quiet, attractive space in a busy high school and its connection to well-being. I need not belabor the point. It is enough to draw attention to "An Afternoon Constitutional," which described the majestic Yale Beinecke Rare Book and Manuscript Library. Its architectural elegance, multi-purpose programming, and openness to the community offer a chance for relaxed reading, intense reflection, and gentle interaction with others. The performance I mentioned was presented by a university group specializing in Renaissance music. The activity punctuated a day of academic activity, offered an opportunity to widen one's horizons, and provided a clear possibility of exploring how others spend their leisure time. It might have offered something special to Nicole and her surroundings in the Paris bistro.

The Beinecke Library reinforces several other points worth mention. First, this library specializes in rare books and manuscripts, which emphasize the need to retain memories of the past and to execute ways of archiving information. I discussed this point in the column on "Archiving Our Pasts," where I suggested that individual and family archiving may contribute to the development and strengthening of identity and belonging. This evokes the use of collecting, pulling memories together through photography and accumulating articles of different types. Memories of cuisine and food also contribute to the habits of home and workspaces, reinforcing the suggestion of permanence and rootedness.

I close this chapter with brief mention of the column "C.L.R. James's *Beyond a Boundary.*" James first published that intriguing text in 1963, and it has remained in the upper echelon of superb sports books. It is true that it is about cricket, a game known well throughout the British Commonwealth. It is also about the life of a Black Trinidadian who used the sport as a lens for examining and exploring cricket, which was a mechanism used by the British to colonize many countries. There is indeed a boundary around every cricket pitch that demarcates where the field of play ends. James wants us to understand that the game of cricket takes place on the field within the boundary. Still, what took place outside the field—where the colonizer was in charge—always found its way onto the field. The compromises required of him in daily life could not be forgotten when he traversed the boundary and entered the field. To do so, he explained, would have required him to change his skin. Thus, as James (1963/1993, p. 66) described it, "the clash of race, caste and class did not retard but stimulated West Indian cricket." Although cricket became a game, a sport like any other, it could readily be transformed into a space that embodied performance, conflict, and resistance. Thus, within every match, an ongoing dialogue exists among the players and between the teams, a representational exchange. This cricket narrative reminds us that the concept of place is not just a theme of geography and architecture. It can also be a stimulus for contemplating ideas, concepts, culture, cuisine, spirituality, and a host of other practices.

## Questions to Ponder

1. Have you considered where you work as a distinctive space with definable characteristics and understandable human interactions?
2. Is there, in your home, a space that you consider the one most conducive to therapeutic activity?
3. Can you describe two or three habits, repeated rituals, that define your home-space and contribute to making it your home?
4. Are there specific things you do to make outsiders welcome in your home?
5. Is food a contributor to the defining of your home-space?

## References

Arkenberg R: Music in the Renaissance, in Heillbrunn Timeline of Art History. New York, Metropolitan Museum of Art, 2000–, October 2002. Available at: http://www.metmuseum.org/toah/hd/renm/hd_renm.htm. Accessed September 6, 2024.

Czepiel K: The art of craft. The Daily Nutmeg New Haven, June 14, 2019

Fullilove MD: Root Shock: How Tearing Up City Neighborhoods Hurts America and What We Can Do About It. New York, Ballantine Books, 2004

Gesler WM: Therapeutic landscapes: medical issues in light of the new cultural geography. Soc Sci Med 34(7):735–746, 1992

Griffith EEH: Race and Excellence: My Dialogue With Chester Pierce. Iowa City, University of Iowa Press, 1998

Griffith EEH: Belonging, Therapeutic Landscapes, and Networks: Implications for Mental Health Practice. New York, Routledge, 2018

Herzog C: Raconte-moi ta vieillesse: tous les jours, je vais au café. Le Monde, June 2, 2024

James CLR: Beyond a Boundary (1963). Durham, NC, Duke University Press, 1993

Liamputtong P, Suwankhong D: Therapeutic landscapes and living with breast cancer: the lived experiences of Thai women. Soc Sci Med 128:263–271, 2015

Livni E: The Japanese practice of 'forest bathing' is scientifically proven to improve your health. Quartz, October 12, 2016

Rowe M: Citizenship and Mental Health. New York, Oxford University Press, 2015

Smyth F: Medical geography: therapeutic places, spaces and networks. Prog Hum Geogr 29(4):488–495, 2005

Walcott D: The Prodigal. New York, Farrar, Straus & Giroux, 2004

# 7

# Seeking Freedom Through the Arts

# Columns From *Psychiatric News*

## Visibility in a Psychiatric Hospital's Museum[1]

I wished long ago that J. K. Rowling had permitted Harry Potter to sell me his invisibility cloak. Then I could have made myself or others invisible or visible at will. Lacking that magical power, many of us simply turn to spending energy, time, and resources trying to render visible those whom we favor and render invisible others who, for one reason or another, confound us.

On a visit to a Caribbean island, I toured a beautifully restored plantation house. The guide took me from a medium-sized bedroom through a door with a latch on it into a smaller area, just barely large enough for a single occupant. The guide asked me to guess how this inner alcove was used, but I was stumped. It turned out to be where the owner sequestered a relative who had a psychiatric illness.

In earlier days, some families preferred this type of physical control of an individual suffering from these illnesses. The explanation was that while the patient was rendered invisible to outsiders, it was a way of keeping the patient safe and protected from untoward events like teasing and accidents. Hospitalization in a psychiatric facility was costly in terms of stigma and its own form of invisibility. The plan of action was often reconsidered if the patient repeated violent behavior or otherwise embarrassed the family.

Despite this history of rendering psychiatric patients invisible, transformative progress continues. Organized efforts have focused on attempts to normalize community living for individuals with psychiatric illness and enhance their access to the privileges of citizenship.

I toured an art exposition at Paris's Sainte-Anne Psychiatric Hospital that ended last month. Titled *Rien à voir: Quand la création échappe au symptôme* (*Nothing to See: When Creation Escapes Symptoms*), the presentation christens the new status of the hospital's art collection as formally a "Musée de France." Thus, the history of this psychiatric hospital and the artistic designs of a cross-section of its patients are now under formal protection in the vast French museum system, under the title of

---

[1] Adapted with permission from Griffith EEH: Visibility in a Psychiatric Hospital's Museum. *Psychiatric News*, January 2020. Copyright © 2020 American Psychiatric Association. All rights reserved.

the Musée d'Art et d'Histoire de l'Hôpital Sainte-Anne. This exposition and the act of creating a national museum in a public hospital form a unique landscape. In it, the hospital's patients can see the possibility of their being artists.

The exposition introduces visitors to 13 artists who painted their works between 1960 and 1970. Anne-Marie Dubois, author of the explanatory text (carrying the same title as the exposition) and the exposition's curator, dives directly into the heart of the matter. How do we look at these paintings done by people who obviously have had significant experience with psychiatric illness? What about the old-time labels ("l'art des fous," "les productions artistiques des maladies mentaux," "l'art brut")?

Dubois reminds us that psychiatrists joined the debate, too, and between 1945 and 1950 conjured up the label of "l'art psychopathologique." This was to make the point that the painters' aesthetic productions were linked to their psychopathology. That statement, for me, reverts to the theme often repeated in recent years about whether people should be defined and limited by their illness. I expect the debate, especially linked to art, will continue.

I include in this column, with the museum's permission, a photograph of the painting used as the thematic reference point of the exposition. It is an untitled piece done by Toubal in 1967 (Figure 7.1). Her first name is unknown, and the work was discovered during an inventory of the hospital's reserve collection. It is possible to conclude that she had spent time as a patient in the hospital, but little else. However, she serves well as a catalyst for the questions raised by Dubois. Are the paintings in the museum documents of psychopathology only to be studied? Or may they also be aesthetic objects, a form of art? And are the artists not free to make of their creativity what they wish? I certainly noticed their celebrity and enhanced visibility.

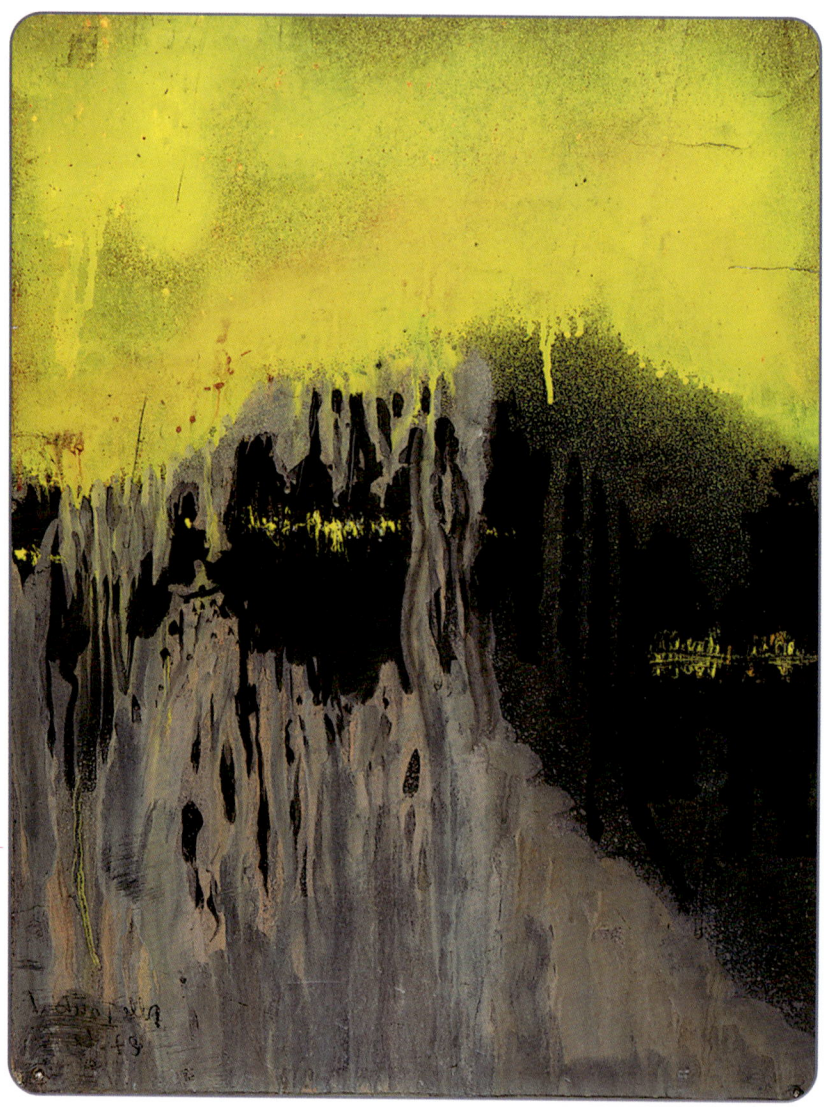

**Figure 7.1** Untitled, 1967, by Toubal.

Gouache on paper.

*Source.* MAHHSA, Musée d'Art et d'Histoire de l'Hôpital Sainte-Anne, Paris. Copyright © Dominique Baliko.

## Stress in Athletes' Lives[2]

In recent months, there has been intense discussion about the connection between competitive sport and mental health. The commentary, focused in large part on the stress endured by elite athletes, has coincided with major international sports events. We have had, almost in back-to-back fashion, the French Open tennis tournament, the Tour de France cycling event, the European 2020 soccer championship, and the Olympics in Japan. Naomi Osaka, a world-famous tennis champion, made the news because of her unwillingness to face the pressure of yet another news conference at the French Open. Some bystanders thought she should respect her obligation to face the public because she had committed to doing so. Others agreed the journalists were offensive. At the Tokyo Olympics, Simone Biles, the American star gymnast, evoked similar conflicting responses when she withdrew from events, citing health matters.

At the European soccer championship, France was eliminated by Switzerland. The match went into overtime and then to a penalty shootout. Kylian Mbappé, a superstar for France, missed his penalty. That outcome sent France's players to the showers and home in disgrace. Mbappé apparently apologized to his fans for what sports writers called a failure. More sympathetic supporters urged him to keep his head up, as the day after the match would mark the debut of a new season. The three athletes I have mentioned illustrate well the stress of competitive athletics.

We follow elite athletes and how they fare on the different terrains of performance. Their annual income and lifestyle, especially in major sports, always attract our attention. Their bodies and minds serve as models of biomedical wonderment for physicians like us. Their capacity for concentration, the sacrifices they make, and their commitment teach us much about what they endure daily.

There are other features of sports that put excitement in our lives. Some years ago, my hospital organized a tournament of bed racing. We closed a street. Different divisions in the facility took a bed, decorated it, named it, and oiled its wheels. An employee, not weighing too much, volunteered to ride in the bed. A team of amateur athletic runners pushed each bed. We all spread the word about the event. The bed-race tournament was on. Every bed had its supporters. I was amazed at how much organized effort was put into this event. We had so much

---

[2] Adapted with permission from Griffith EEH: Stress in Athletes' Lives. *Psychiatric News*, October 2021. Copyright © 2021 American Psychiatric Association. All rights reserved.

fun that I forgot to ask where the idea had originated. Athletics, competition, and team spirit came together and reawakened the slumbering youth in all of us, even in the bystanders.

With these wonderfully positive notions about competitive sports so present in our culture, how did the idea take root that elite athletes are the very incarnation of perfection and are obliged to meet public expectations? We must know that they make mistakes from time to time in what they do, and anxiety haunts the best of them. While performances may be breathtaking, consistently flawless performance is hard to sustain. So, why this mourning and weeping over the mistakes of our athletes and their inability to cope well with stress at every event? Why not just console and encourage them when they are facing loss, injury, and disappointing performances?

I still recall the early years in elementary school running after a soccer ball on the playground without quite knowing what to do with it. Eventually, the running was accompanied by thoughtful preparation and strategy. I remember the contentment of belonging to a group, the sense of accomplishment, learning about leadership when I captained the team, feeling the admiration of bystanders when I scored a goal. I also learned about losing in the context of competition and about the pain of a torn muscle during excessive effort.

We should urge sports enthusiasts to stop pretending that the elite athlete owes them continual brilliant performances. We should remonstrate with coaches who never prepare a substitute for the day that the star center forward on the soccer team will be unable to play. We know that sports can be pleasurable enough to evoke a kind of loyalty from fans that borders on spiritual commitment. We recognize sports' service as an antidote to the drudgery of daily life. Still, creating an idealistic vision of athletics misleads us all. There is risk in the act of living, and that includes sports.

# A Flamenco Tale in Edinburgh: Recreating Home[3]

The Edinburgh Festival is well known, but I was never able to attend it until this past summer. I made the most of the occasion and immersed myself in several simple and fabulous productions. I liked

---

[3] Adapted with permission from Griffith EEH: A Flamenco Tale in Edinburgh: Recreating Home. *Psychiatric News*, December 2021. Copyright © 2021 American Psychiatric Association. All rights reserved.

## Seeking Freedom Through the Arts

the one-woman musical play *Black Is the Color of My Voice*, about the life of the American singer and pianist Nina Simone. The performance of African music by Sona Jobarteh on the Kora, a 21-string Gambian instrument, was spellbinding. A flamenco concert of song and dance led by the Spanish guitarist Daniel Martinez completed this trilogy of differentiated works of art that verified for me the meaning of an arts festival. The three productions conjured up the connection to geography and migration. They told stories of the relationship of art and the movements of daily life. With a bit of imagination while viewing these performances, one could create narratives of loss, cultural displacement, love, and triumphant reengagement.

The flamenco concert was a more personal experience, as the venue was smaller and more intimate than the others. At the close of the production, I was able to chat with Daniel Martinez, the 28-year-old guitarist and leader of his own flamenco company in Scotland. My first question focused on the meaning of his production's title, "Art of Believing." Before answering, he explained that he grew up in the Spanish city of Cordova and spent well over a decade training in music theory and performance on the flamenco guitar. He graduated from the Royal Conservatory of Music in Cordova. After years of teaching and gaining professional experience at home in Spain, he participated in a music festival abroad. Then came the idea of leaving home, spreading his wings, and thinking about putting roots down in another country. He concluded that he could solidify his artistic identity in a foreign country where he could tell others about his music and share it. The production title was a way of displaying belief in himself, the music, and the commitment to his culture and antecedents.

The performance that evening was delivered by Daniel Martinez on guitar; Danielo Olivera and Inma Montero, both obviously adept at the flamenco chanson; and Gabriela Pouso, a flamenco dancer of the first order (Figure 7.2). They played off each other in turn, then in unison, and at other times produced remarkable solos. They served, too, as members of a harmonic chorus by singing, clapping, and stamping feet. Moods changed, reflecting tales of betrayal and disappointment, then stories of attachment and contentment. The dancer's movements described passion, funereal regret, invitations to the fortunate, and disgust at the treachery of others. The handclapping was executed crisply and clearly in the group celebrations. The flamenco clap often uses that intertwining of the thumbs as the hands come together. The sound is sharp and explicitly rhythmic. All this continued as the guitarist expertly guided the dramatic storytelling with his music and

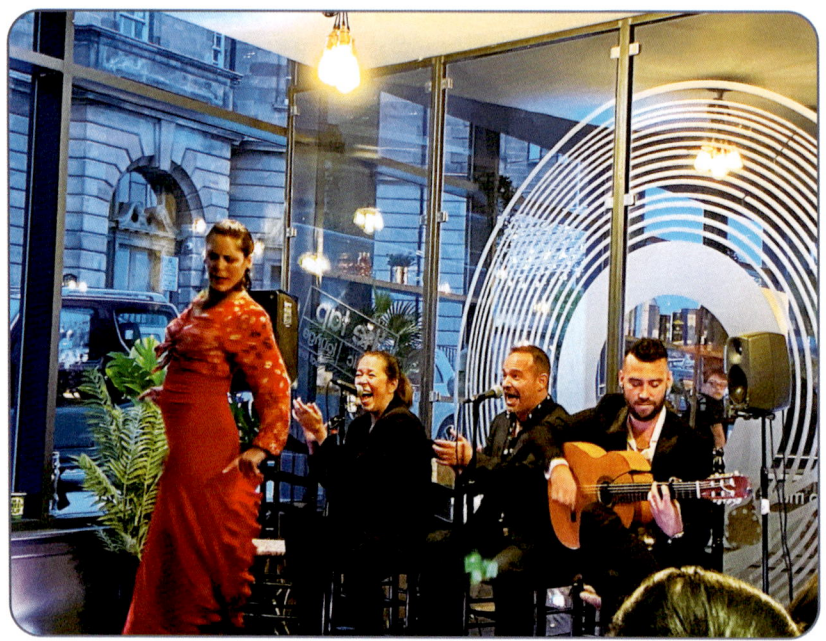

**Figure 7.2** A Flamenco Celebration in Edinburgh, United Kingdom.

Flamenco dancer Gabriela Pouso performs with musicians from the Daniel Martinez Flamenco Company at the Edinburgh Festival.

*Source.* Photograph by Brigitte Griffith, with permission from Daniel Martinez Flamenco Company.

punctuation. There was always the sense of fundamental community in the small group of performers, which extended to the audience.

Some scholars see flamenco as the folkloric music traditions of the Andalusian region of Spain, powerfully influenced by the Gitanos, or Gypsies, who migrated from Egypt across India in the 15th century and ended up in Spain. Claims are made, too, about a connection between flamenco music and early peasant songs. Others note the influence of Islamic, Jewish, and African culture in the music. *Flamenco* may well be an Arabic word, some say. The opening of 19th-century cafés and bars (cafés cantantes), hosting flamenco singing and dancing, is thought to have cemented the popularity of this new wave in Spain's cultural landscape.

The performance of the Daniel Martinez Flamenco Company resurrected for me the challenge of recreating home outside its conventional boundary. Every year, some of us pursue this desire to move elsewhere.

We do it while confronting the problems inherent in self-exile from our home countries. We somehow manage to transform the probable danger into renewed opportunity as we refashion and improve our lives. Here, I am speaking of voluntary migration. Making the journey under duress is another matter altogether. The Daniel Martinez Company illustrated the possibility of drawing life from art. I could feel freedom in the music, dance, and song. As the famous artist Josef Albers suggested, art informs us about seeing and feeling life, and music carries life inside itself. The dance company made that point, and I understood better the art of believing.

## Yonder on the Other Side[4]

Paris is a beautiful and beguiling city. Visitors must be careful about reacting too quickly to the city's obvious charm and seduction. I recently attended a Paris performance of Claudio Monteverdi's *1610 Vespers* (*Vêpres de la Vierge*) at the modern auditorium of the stunning Radio France building. A few days later, I was listening to lectures at the Quai Branly Jacques Chirac Museum on the artistic culture of Bénin, formerly the French colony of Dahomey. Such experiences in quick succession induce relaxation, intellectual stimulation, and enjoyment of the surrounding aesthetics. However, sustaining that state of mind is hard.

I am sitting one evening in a small theater watching a play, *Là-Bas de L'Autre Côté de L'Eau* (*Yonder on the Other Side of the Water*), written by Pierre Olivier Scotto and directed by Xavier Lemaire. The scene is French Algeria in the 1950s. Enter France, an attractive and lively young woman who is enamored of things French. She is in love with Moktar, a vibrant Algerian militant—that is, until a young French soldier shows up on the scene and gets France's head and heart spinning. France's mother, Marthe, whose husband died at the hands of French soldiers, is not pleased about her daughter's new love interest. I knew immediately that we were on sensitive ground. Algeria is always a dangerous subject when one is in Paris.

William Gardner Smith's newly republished book, *The Stone Face* (1963/2021), comes to mind. Smith first published the book in 1963 and focused on the experience of Black Americans exiling themselves to

---

[4] Adapted with permission from Griffith EEH: Yonder on the Other Side. *Psychiatric News*, January 2022. Copyright © 2022 American Psychiatric Association. All rights reserved.

Paris around that time to flee the racism in the United States. An important theme in the book is the discovery by the main protagonist of a puzzling contradiction. The French welcomed the Black American exiles while venting wrath on the Algerians, who were at the bottom of the country's caste system. James Hannaham (2021) highlighted the significance of these anti-Arab sentiments when he reviewed Smith's book.

The Algerian War (1954–1962) is the setting for the play. The Algerian National Liberation Front (NLF) wants independence from France. However, there is a constituency of French Algerians, including Marthe, demanding that the mother country stay the course, keep the colony, and maintain French identity. In the mid-1950s, the independence movement heated up with significant violence. The NLF placed its bombs in Paris and at home with terrifying effect. The French authorities responded firmly and matched terror with their own brand. The Paris Massacre of October 17, 1961 (referenced in Smith's book), saw policemen throwing NLF demonstrators into the Seine River, causing the death of hundreds. On October 17, 2019, this event was memorialized by the construction of a stele, a monument with an inscription, placed at the Saint-Michel Bridge that crosses the Seine (Figure 7.3).

French and Algerians had been living side by side for years. Algerians served in the French Army and fought in World War II. However, the French government would not pay pensions to Algerian veterans, although French veterans were compensated. Each side had its grievances. Moktar, too, is caught in the violence. He wants the French out of Algeria. The trouble with that simple demand is that many French Algerians have never set foot in France; France is not their home. The audience understands that finding a solution to the conflict is not easy.

By the end of the play, we know that there can be no obvious triumph for anybody. There is a claim that personal identity has been clarified and solidified for some. Young France must put limits on her imagination. The French Republic recognizes, long after the war, that promises were broken to both sides. Many people died in the Algerian conflict.

There are always observers who insist that violence is the only way to overturn the caste ladder. The water between Algeria and France does not magically wash away memories and judgments of the other. If we are not careful, those recollections stoke the fire of vengeance. The path to reconciliation is uncomfortable, not pleasurable like listening to Monteverdi. Nevertheless, the play is a beautiful experience, even if heartrending, to witness dramatic art confronting struggles related to colonization, caste, indignity, and freedom of spirit.

*Seeking Freedom Through the Arts*

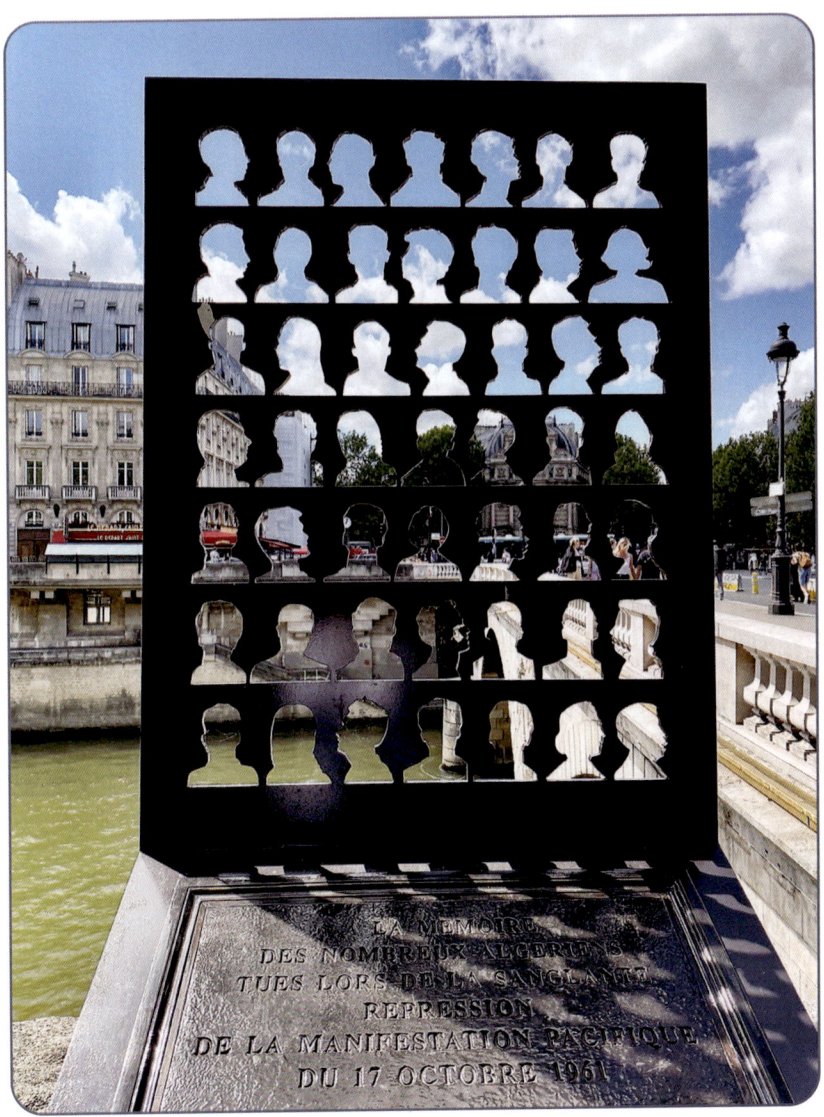

**Figure 7.3**  Public Monument on the Seine River, Paris, France.

This sculpture memorializes the death of Algerian National Liberation Front fighters in the Paris Massacre of 1961.

*Source.*   Photograph by Brigitte Griffith.

## The Solitude of an Artist[5]

It was a rainy October evening, with no promise of a respite. So, I accepted the comfort of an invitation indoors to watch a play. The theater was a local Parisian space comfortably seating about 200 individuals. The play, *Glenn: Naissance d'un Prodige* (*Glenn: Birth of a Prodigy*), was written by Ivan Calbérac. It is the story of the famous Glenn Gould, considered one of the greatest pianists of the 20th century. He is celebrated mainly as an interpreter of Johann Sebastian Bach's piano compositions. Other observers have described his talents as a writer, composer, and conductor; however, the play, obviously pursuing condensation of his life story, focused on the development of his skills on the pianoforte.

He was born in Canada on September 25, 1932, and died on October 4, 1982. Reports describe his childhood exposure to music and the involvement of his mother in his piano lessons. His possession of perfect pitch, a phenomenal musical memory, and an exquisitely attentive mother all played a part in his success. He enrolled in the Royal Conservatory of Music in Toronto, Ontario, at age 10 and apparently passed his final Conservatory examination on that instrument at age 12.

We learned early in the play that Gould's mother followed through on her lessons. She sometimes restricted him to a closet for having misidentified a note. He had difficulty falling asleep, which caused her to schedule nights for her to sleep in his bed and calm him. There was a dramatic scene in which she and his father argued about the excessive time she slept at her son's side. Father advised her that it was not a good practice. She dismissed this silly talk and highlighted her commitment to promoting her son's artistry.

This maternal devotion is portrayed in different ways by Calbérac. Mother protects her son from the natural intrusions of mundane life, such as the inevitable encounters with female friends. When the telephone rings, she answers and finds creative excuses for Glenn's unavailability. She does not hide her actions as much as she argues to herself that such relationships take time away from the central task of preparing a performing artist.

As Calbérac frames the events, this mother-son interaction becomes legitimately two-sided. It comes into full view toward the end of the play when his mother, at age 83, is hospitalized and near death. He

---

[5] Adapted with permission from Griffith EEH: The Solitude of an Artist. *Psychiatric News*, December 2022. Copyright © 2022 American Psychiatric Association. All rights reserved.

wants to see her and cannot bring himself to do it. After all, going to the hospital may bring him in contact with germs and cause him to have, yes, a nosocomial infection. That has been a major fear much of his life, one that led to his wearing gloves and not shaking hands with people. Unsurprisingly, then, when she dies, he chastises himself as an ungrateful son for denying her the pleasure of seeing him at the end. He did not make the trip to see this woman who had given so much of herself to making him comfortable and a successful artist.

In the informal debriefing after the performance, some friends mused that this mother had gotten what she certainly expected from an alexithymic son. She must have understood that her son had complicated ways of expressing his emotions toward people. That assumes he possessed feelings about individuals. Little proof crops up in the play supporting this. In fact, it is hard to define what he feels about that other woman, aside from his mother, the one who followed him dutifully for years, waiting for a sign of love or even of acknowledgment that she was loyal to him.

Having 50 years to cover in this prodigy's life story, the playwright takes on the major task of highlighting a few features of Gould's experiences. No psychological terms are used—just the provision of evidence in snippets. Gould has an exceptional memory for the language of music. While he lacks easy connections to people, he has a deep emotional relation with music. For example, when I listen to his piano playing, I remark easily how his execution of a few bars of music is so profoundly dynamic. Notes that are of equal duration and volume become performatively distinct, varied, like the way we speak. Monotony disappears. It becomes clear that he is playing something he hears, not what is written on the sheet. This insistence on the enveloped self within the music emerges in the idea that he wished to control the product of each performance. On stage, there was the discussion about his wanting to direct every aspect of the music. This effectively resulted in his withdrawal from public concerts. He preferred delivering nonaudience recitals in his recordings; he described the audience as torture. Public performance had become torture.

This produced a form of isolation in everyday life that starts with his body—in the closet and later wrapped in winter clothing and gloves, even in summer. There is, too, the withdrawal from community and family. There is a scene in which his agent resigns, and Gould asks him to stay. The representative points out that there is nothing for him to do. Everything is set up to run like clockwork. But Gould wants him to hang around, just not too close. Anthropologists talk of socialities, of our need for each other, of the pressing interrelatedness of human beings. This prodigy lived it differently.

## Seeking Nirvana at the Potter's Wheel[6]

It is one thing to see visual artists' productions in a museum, disconnected from the artists. It is a different experience to talk to them directly and intimately about their work. I recently spent about a month with 80-year-old Ronald Grantham, AIA, visiting museums in France and discussing different aspects of his pottery. I had come to know him over several generations because of interfamily linkages. He is an architect who established his distinguished reputation over 35 years on the staff of Connecticut architect Warren Platner.

Ron's primary interest has always been the designing of buildings and interiors. Concerning the passion for design work, he explained that "Everything I look at I'm trying to make it look better." One of his first love affairs was with Frank Lloyd Wright's Fallingwater, which was a home designed by Wright. It was built in 1936 in Mill Run, Pennsylvania. In his youth, Ron felt an urge to emulate Wright's work. Once Ron retired from the practice of architecture around 2012, he returned to pottery, something he had started years before, during his architectural training at California State Polytechnic University.

He grew up in the San Francisco, California, area in the 1940s with two siblings. While his mother painted all the time, she and he rarely engaged in deep conversations about art. Still, she encouraged his drawing. Her influence evidently got through to him, as he recalls readily that he enjoyed drawing but did not use color. He was attracted to mechanical drawing classes in high school. In one such class, around 1958, he learned about a contest sponsored by the East Bay Women's Architectural League. The project task was to design a house for a specific number of occupants and deliver a floor plan, exterior elevations, and a three-dimensional view. He described this activity, noting that he really did not have enough experience to ensure a chance of winning the competition. Still, he never gave up, and with minimal supervision he finished the project. Although he did not win the contest,

---

[6] Adapted with permission from Griffith EEH: Seeking Nirvana at the Potter's Wheel. *Psychiatric News*, February 2023. Copyright © 2023 American Psychiatric Association. All rights reserved.

the experience brought an inner feeling of confidence that he would become an architect.

He obtained his architecture university degree in 1968 and spent a year preparing for the first part of his licensure examinations. He also married his college sweetheart at this time. Then he fulfilled his commitment to the military, serving a 2-year stint as an officer in the U.S. Army Corps of Engineers. After discharge, he studied photography for a year, then moved to Connecticut to take up a position with Warren Platner's firm. It was in this job that he saw his professional skills develop and his creative interests flourish. Ron explained that Platner certainly had his own ideas. However, as a supervisor, Platner also encouraged his staff to indulge their own passions and defend them in open discussions. In this relationship with another artist-architect, Ron participated in the designs of restaurants (such as Windows on the World in New York City), hotels, offices, and private residences.

Ron's return to pottery during his retirement marked the beginning of personal reflection about his development as a ceramist. He initially worked on bowls and cups, producing what he describes as semi-utilitarian objects. He was not satisfied with the results. Then he moved on to working with white porcelain that obviates use of a glaze. The emphasis on three-dimensional shapes progressively took root. He wanted to emphasize purity of form and experimented with bending the shapes and polishing the form to smoothness. He avoided texture and use of color. Nowadays, he likes playing with curves and voids, developing contrasts within a single object.

The photograph (Figure 7.4) represents his present work. It is a 12-inch-high white sculpture whose primary design element is the spherical shape. The second design element incorporates vertical curves on the right side, reinforced by the smaller curves visible on the top. A contrasting element is the vertical edge on the left side of the opening. The finger lines running horizontally on the inside reinforce the spherical shape of the structure. The white color additionally forces concentration on the three-dimensional form. It is worth mentioning that Ron signs his work with a simple letter R placed on the outside bottom of the work, to avoid encroachment on the design objective.

He states plainly that his focus is on art for its own sake. He distills satisfaction that is bereft of sociopolitical content. He likes the freedom embodied in the conceptualization and execution of his sculptures. He experiences a variety of emotions in the creative act. But he does not wish the work itself to contain any message from him, although he concedes that he has no control over what a viewer sees in the finished

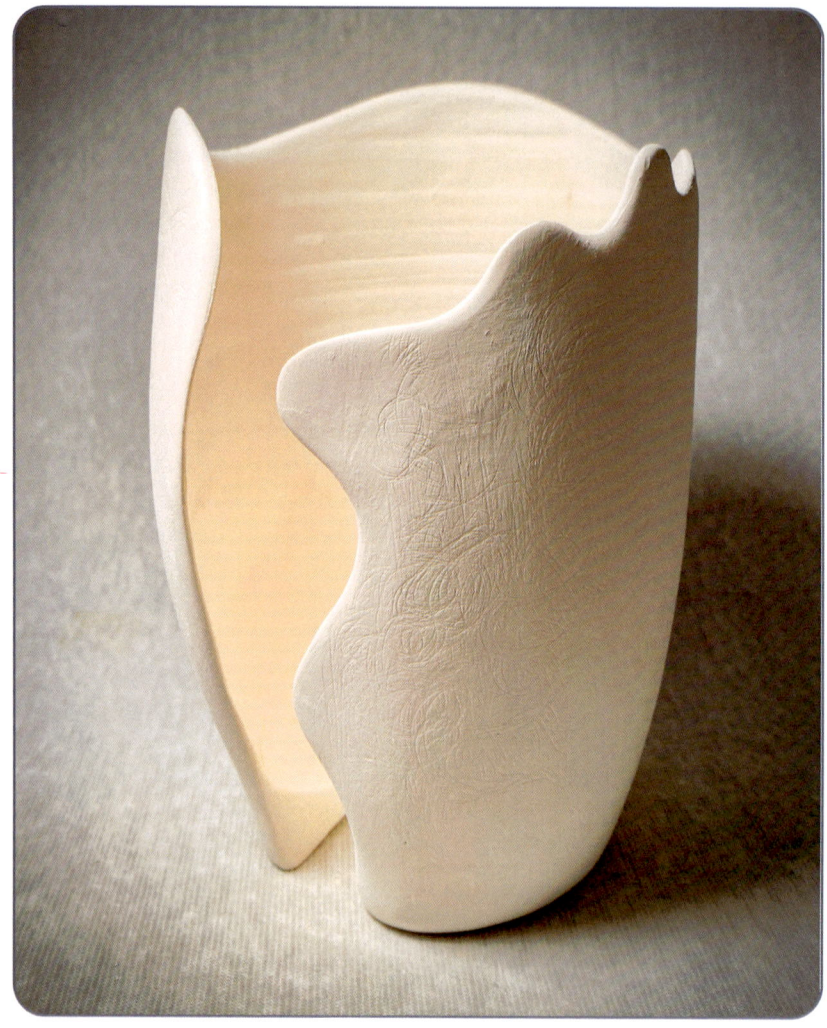

**Figure 7.4** *Bajan Wave* by R. C. Grantham, AIA.

Celebrating art for art's sake.

*Source.* Private Anonymous Collection. Used with permission. Photograph by R. C. Grantham, AIA.

product. He takes no responsibility for the viewer's meaning-making. He revels in his personal freedom to contribute to the beauty around us. He can also understand the privilege the artist has in the formulation of aesthetics. I challenge him, saying that he certainly has charted a different route from, for example, Jean-Michel Basquiat, Henri Matisse, or

Claude Monet. These are some of the many artists we have discussed recently. He eschews such comparisons. He is pleased with the palpable peacefulness and beauty of his work, with its distance from any social movement. He represents himself.

## Ancestral Dignity in Public Monuments[7]

Some months ago, I wrote a column about the removal of Lord Horatio Nelson's (1758–1805) statue from a public square in Barbados. The political decision to uproot artistic evidence of the country's long history of being colonized had generated much commentary throughout the island about dignity and identity. I ended the column with a reference to the Caribbean Nobel winner Derek Walcott, who had chastised Caribbean peoples for their envy of European statues and had urged them to contemplate the beauty of the Caribbean and other matters more relevant to their modern lives.

In my most recent trip to Barbados, just about everybody urged me to visit the Golden Square Freedom Park. It was obvious that the creation of the park was an event that had galvanized a return to families and friends interrogating themselves about their roots, the meaning of their country's independence from colonial masters, and who and what should be celebrated. Nelson was not even an afterthought in any of these discussions. I learned that in 1999, the Ministry of Education and Culture commissioned a group to develop a project that would celebrate individuals who had contributed to the island's overall development. From my discussions, I understood this to include "unsung heroes" like the Amerindians who had inhabited the island before the arrival of the first British settlers, the indentured servants who were members of the island's labor force, and the African enslaved persons and their descendants who had made contributions to the island's progress.

The 2-acre park rests a stone's throw away from the site previously occupied by the Nelson statue in Bridgetown, the capital city. The park's inauguration occurred on November 29, 2021, a day before the island's transformation into a parliamentary republic. We should remember that Barbados became independent from Great Britain on November 30, 1966. It is with these dates in mind that I reflected on

---

[7] Adapted with permission from Griffith EEH: Ancestral Dignity in Public Monuments. *Psychiatric News*, April 2023. Copyright © 2023 American Psychiatric Association. All rights reserved.

friends' urging me to visit the new space. Many of them were enthusiastic about describing their impressions and providing background information. Construction of the Freedom Park required demolition of several buildings that previously occupied the site. Not everybody was pleased with the decision.

The Freedom Park was established in a working-class area of Bridgetown, where Clement Payne used to conduct mass meetings in the 1930s urging Black Barbadians to resist the White planter class. Clement Osbourne Payne was born in Trinidad to Barbadian parents in 1904. His parents apparently returned to Barbados with their young son around 1908. He progressively earned a reputation in Barbados as a trade unionist and advocate of social justice, especially after spending more time in late-1920s Trinidad sharpening his militancy. He was opposed by the White landowners and ultimately deported from Barbados on July 26, 1937, following the riots provoked by his political agitating. The statue of Clement Payne, shown in Figure 7.5, is an important symbol in Freedom Park and is accompanied by another monument nearby. The two make a collective memorial to the individuals who lost their lives or suffered in the struggle for freedom in the 1937 revolt.

The conceptual idea of unsung heroes mentioned earlier was concretized by the creation of the "Builders of Barbados Wall." It is constructed from bricks on which are inscribed Barbadian surnames. The wall, shown in Figure 7.6, celebrates thousands of ordinary people who, although lacking fame or prominence, contributed to the development of Barbados over the past 600 years. Commentators have noted that the monument symbolizes an appreciation of ancestral dignity and illustrates a sense of belonging that everyone hopes can be cultivated in the island's youth. It is considered an interactive method of bringing history to life.

I did visit this new Golden Square Freedom Park. I stood and looked, walked around, and approached strangers to talk about this novel development. Only one man, sitting on a bench absorbed in his private business, gave me a withering look. I left him alone. I watched small groups searching for their names, obviously absorbed in the task of self-recognition, with satisfaction on their faces once the discovery was made. I heard regrets and concerns expressed about the park's proximity to neighborhoods that needed refurbishing. This suggested to observers that the surrounding blight might engulf the park unless maintenance remained a central feature. There was a clear understanding of what some have called a gospel of self-respect, enunciated by

*Seeking Freedom Through the Arts*

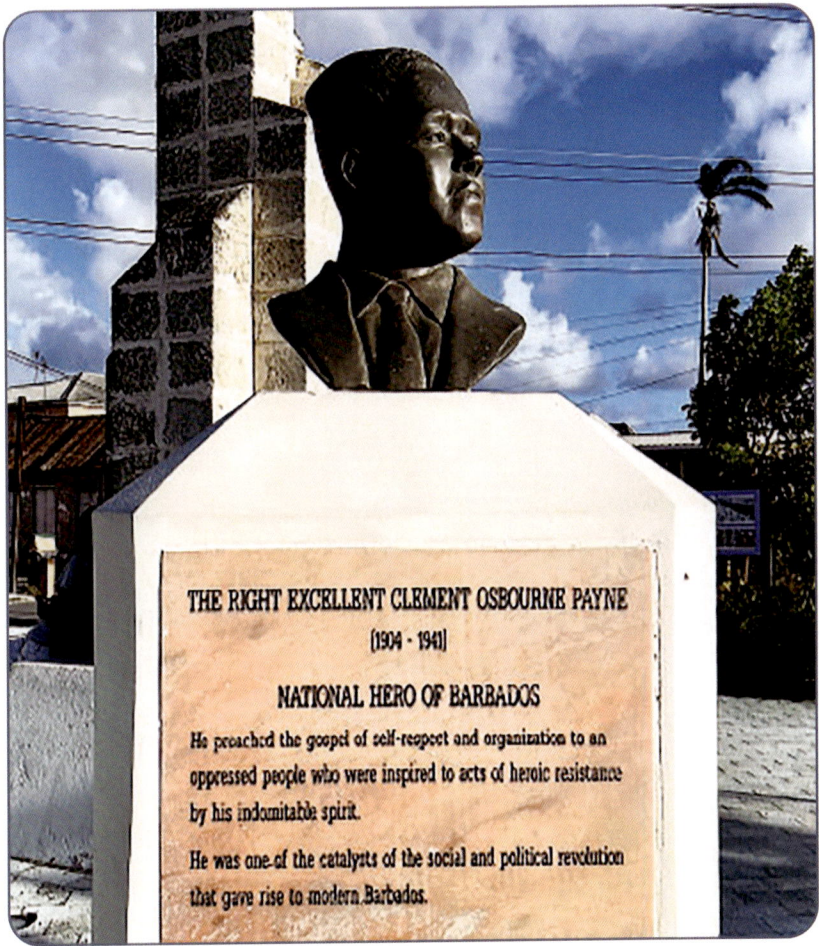

**Figure 7.5** Clement Payne Statue, Barbados.

The public monument honors the trade unionist (1904–1941) who was named a National Hero of Barbados.

*Source.* Photograph by Brigitte Griffith.

Clement Payne. There was talk, too, of the new theme of ancestral dignity evident as families searched for their names on the monument's bricks. Like everybody else, I scrutinized bricks and felt satisfied when I discovered my name in its three Welsh versions: Griffith, Griffiths, and Griffin. It made me think about what my father and grandfather had contributed to nation building. In any case, they had done more for Barbados than Lord Nelson.

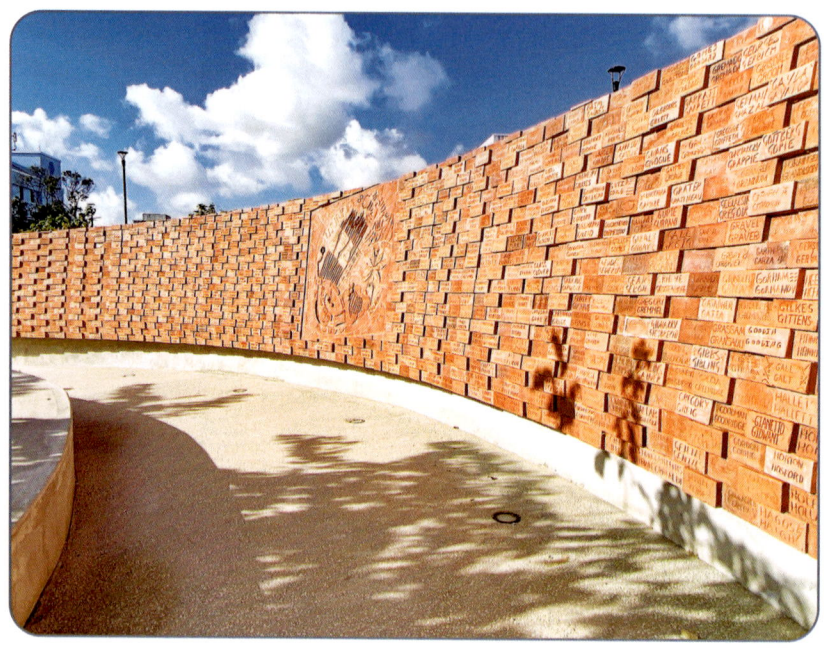

**Figure 7.6** Builders of Barbados Wall, Barbados.

This structure honors unsung heroes who contributed to the country's development.

*Source.* Photograph by Brigitte Griffith.

## Talkin' 'Bout Harlem[8]

There has been much talk about *The Harlem Renaissance and Transatlantic Modernism*, a current exhibit at The Metropolitan Museum of Art (The Met) on New York City's Fifth Avenue. With the breadth and intensity of the advertising, I had to witness this event directly. The show was clearly a landmark happening on the broad cultural scene as well as in the world of American art.

Regardless of the debates in this country about race matters, the exhibit's visitors on the day I attended were diverse in all sorts of ways. Grandmothers explained images to their grandchildren. White, Black, and Brown people exchanged friendly glances and patiently waited in

---

[8] Adapted with permission from Griffith EEH: Talkin' 'Bout Harlem. *Psychiatric News*, July 2024. Copyright © 2024 American Psychiatric Association. All rights reserved.

turn to examine a piece of art. I finally gave up counting the different languages being spoken around me. Dignity was in the air, and self-satisfaction was engraved on many faces. The entire scene illustrated the notion of curiosity about the other, something that psychiatrists usually find so hard to explain.

Allison Meier (2024), writing in *The Art Newspaper*, pointed out that in 1969, at the same museum, the exhibit *Harlem on My Mind* opened without including any Black painters or sculptors. Critics noted that talking about Harlem while disregarding "the pivotal role of artists in the activism and community of Harlem" made little sense. It represented an insidious form of segregation. Holland Cotter (2024), in "The Met Aims to Get Harlem Right, the Second Time Around," mentioned that there was apparently considerable picketing around The Met at the time by a group of contemporary artists who demanded inclusion and affirmation of their cultural identity, "in art as in life." Cotter noted that while The Met did not frame the current exhibit as an "institutional correction," one could characterize it as "moving a still-neglected art history out of the wings and onto the main stage." In 1987, things were better at the Studio Museum of Harlem's show called *Harlem Renaissance: Art of Black America*, curated by Mary Campbell and David Driskell. The catalogue, edited by Charles Miers (1987), which accompanied that exhibit, offers a helpful summary of the Harlem Renaissance movement.

Cotter (2024) referred to the Harlem Renaissance as running roughly from 1918 through the 1930s. There is fluidity about this conceptualization, as artists working outside that period are mentioned in relation to the movement. Not all of them lived in Harlem, and neither was the movement considered only a visual art phenomenon. Writers and musicians were included, as well as photographers. That was when, as the curators noted, artists were engaging with Black writers, performers, and composers in what was also called the New Negro movement. Veronica Chambers and Michelle May-Curry (2024) suggested that the Harlem Renaissance represented "a flowering of intellectual and artistic activity that would give the neighborhood and its residents global renown." Three intellectual stalwarts of the time (Alain Locke, W. E. B. Du Bois, and Charles Johnson) are often named as leaders of the movement.

Allison Meier (2024) pointed out that Alain Locke, as the theorist of the Harlem Renaissance, adopted a point of view or ethos concerning the work of Black American artists. Locke wanted them to respect the artistic heritage of Africa, particularly its sculptural tradition. The result, he hoped, would be an authentic African American aesthetic. This intellectualized approach found support among painters and sculptors who were familiar with the European scene. Other Black American artists turned to glorifying the tradition of Black folklore and creating a kind of primitive art form. There were still others who focused on the details of Black life. This latter preoccupation had its own difficulties, as some observers found certain slices of Harlem life difficult to accept. Participants in the Renaissance confronted discrimination on Harlem streets and in their professional lives. There was, too, an active antiracism movement carried out in early 20th-century America by organizations such as the National Association for the Advancement of Colored People (founded in 1909); the Urban League (created in 1910); and Marcus Garvey's United Negro Improvement Association, which was developed toward the end of World War I.

Consequently, the Harlem Renaissance artists were concerned about their own segregated status and with questions of identity. In the introduction to the 1987 museum catalogue, Mary Campbell discussed the Renaissance visual artists' struggle to establish a clear aesthetic identity for themselves. She also considered whether the Black artist could or should be set apart from White colleagues. There was a substantial difference of opinion concerning these matters. David Lewis, writing in the same 1987 museum catalogue, noted that by the mid-1920s, there were some who held the view that art was not principally about politics and race matters, but about genuineness, a form of truth that tends to be in the beholder's eyes.

The debate crystallized around Claude McKay's novel *Home to Harlem* (1928). Lewis stated that as the novel portrayed no one resembling Du Bois or Locke, the Black bourgeoisie considered it unrefined and coarse. Apparently, Du Bois stated that while the novel did not portray Black America's talented tenth, it certainly represented its debauched tenth. The novel had clearly strayed from the rules articulated by the civil rights establishment. The struggle over Black identity had smoldered even as Harlem solidly established itself as "Black America's Paris" in literature, art and sculpture, jazz music, photography, theater, and the social club scene. While the Harlem Renaissance was said to portray racial talent and confidence, the question of Black identity remained the subject of intense debate. The curator Mary Campbell made the point that if the Renaissance artists contributed anything, it was to demonstrate that the Black artist could influence Black American images.

It is this feeling of being in control that often provides the individual, fighting for recognition and independence, a sense of equality. Holland Cotter (2024) suggested that other aspects of the current exhibit point to factors that render the identity search a complex undertaking. There is, for example, the matter of "colorism," hinted at in *Mother and Daughter*, a 1927 painting by Laura Waring. The work points to the existence of a social ladder among Blacks founded on skin color. Beauford Delaney's 1941 nude portrait of a young James Baldwin immediately forces a conversation about sexuality and homophobia. Meta Fuller's sculpture *Mary Turner (A Silent Protest Against Mob Violence)* invites conversation on whether Black artists should be exempted from forced participation in the antiracism movement. Should Black artists allow themselves to be forcibly drafted into the identity politics stand of cultural solidarity?

## Suzanne Césaire and Caribbean Identity[9]

I left home on a rainy Sunday afternoon in late September to view *The Ballad of Suzanne Césaire*, a 16-mm film about the French-Caribbean writer and activist, directed by Madeleine Hunt-Ehrlich and screened as part of the New York Film Festival at Manhattan's Lincoln Center. I was interested because I knew that Suzanne Césaire was the wife of the world-famous Aimé Césaire, a French writer, politician, and public intellectual. However, the film's screenplay emphasizes that the narrative is about her, not him. Commenting on Suzanne Césaire's work in *Diacritik*, Gabrielle Saïd (2016) referred to Césaire's feminine voice hidden in the shadow behind the solar presence of her husband. Suzanne Césaire has also been called the missing mother of the negritude movement, as she never received much recognition for its success.

Film notes circulated at the screening depict Hunt-Ehrlich as a visual artist interested in elucidating hidden parts of Black women's lives. She is concerned that women are often burdened by various gender-based constraints. This partly explains why mere fragments of information exist about Suzanne Césaire's life story, in comparison to her husband's international popularity. Hunt-Ehrlich also thinks that, in general, racist and patriarchal structures limit the public spread of Black female artists' work. As I watched *The Ballad of Suzanne Césaire*,

---

[9] Adapted with permission from Griffith EEH: Suzanne Césaire and Caribbean Identity. *Psychiatric News*, December 2024. Copyright © 2024 American Psychiatric Association. All rights reserved.

I wondered about Hunt-Ehrlich's positionality in relation to the film's subject, especially when it became obvious that she was committed to creating a story about Césaire from mere fragments of a narrative. Hunt-Ehrlich conceded that the task was difficult and Suzanne Césaire well-nigh unknowable.

I was unprepared for a film that so evidently relied on the director's imagination to flesh out the factual fragments of a life. It also took me some time to understand that the production would make use of surrealist imagery to strengthen its storyline. One good illustration is a scene that features an actress reading lines from Suzanne Césaire's work amid a tropical storm. The incongruous juxtaposition of howling winds and rain against the act of reading serious literature evokes Césaire's connection to surrealism. A similar symbolism arises in another scene as the camera focuses on the wind's scattering of sheets of paper that may have represented an unpublished copy of Suzanne Césaire's work. In addition, we see Césaire in the presence of a male figure I identified as André Breton, the leader of surrealism. The tableau, ambiguous and provocative, raises questions about its placement and significance.

So, we have an intriguing cinematic tale built on structural fragments and creative imagination. There are other data available from collateral sources. Suzanne Césaire was born in August 1915 on the Caribbean island of Martinique and died in May 1966 in France. She received her early education on the island and went to France in 1933 to study philosophy and literature, first in Toulouse and then in Paris. From 1936 to 1938, she was a student at the prestigious École Normale Supérieure. During her stay in Paris, she met Léopold Senghor, leader of the famous negritude literary protest movement mentioned earlier, which is said to have been influenced by the Harlem Renaissance of the 1920s and 1930s, especially the work of Langston Hughes and Claude McKay.

Suzanne Césaire also participated in the founding of a journal called *L'Étudiant Noir*, activity considered fundamental preparation for the literary work that she and her husband took up soon after they returned to Martinique in 1939. While in Paris, she married Aimé Césaire and gave birth to the first of their six children. On their return to the Caribbean, both she and her husband held teaching jobs at local high schools while coediting a cultural and literary revue named *Tropiques* with René Ménil and Aristide Maugée. *Tropiques* lasted from 1941 to 1945, and it is in that journal that Suzanne Césaire published seven essays that eventually brought her international fame as a cultural intellectual.

Writing in the *International Journal of Surrealism*, María Bernal (2023) put Suzanne Césaire at the crossroads of surrealism, negritude, and French Caribbean decolonization. Bernal maintains that it was a critical event in 1941 when a cargo ship docked in Fort-de-France with André Breton, Claude Lévi-Strauss, and others who were fleeing war and persecution in Europe. The encounter between artists and writers of the Caribbean and Europe led to the surrealists' agreement to join forces with the Martiniquans in their anticolonial struggle. Bernal notes that scholars have discussed this meeting, while saying little about Suzanne Césaire's obvious contribution.

Bernal also points out that Aimé Césaire and René Ménil had a strong interest in cultivating a political role connected to Martinique's future status in relation to France. They were politicians. On the other hand, Suzanne Césaire wanted to transform the psychology of the Martiniquan population, many of whom had adopted assimilation as their acculturative response to France. She wanted to restore her people's lost identity with something authentically Black, but not rooted in Africa. No! As Kara Rabbitt (2008) framed it in the journal *Research in African Literatures*, Césaire wanted to emphasize place not origin. She had enough of Africa as a source of mythic beginnings. She was seeking self-acknowledgment. She had confidence in the generational continuity derived from three centuries of contact with the land and people of Martinique.

There was, of course, instability in this new Martiniquan identity. But no matter! It was, for her, grounded in the Antilles, her land. Among the fragments in *The Ballad of Suzanne Césaire* are links to African drums and negritude, as well as connections to France and to European intellectuals (including Freud). However, Rabbitt confirms that Suzanne Césaire was looking to her freedom as a Martiniquan woman. Césaire also resented the vision of Martinique as a bucolic land waiting to give pleasure submissively. She was interested in political power acquired through generations of women and resting on a new cultural authenticity and recognition of self.

## Comments and Clinical Observations

It was a remarkable piece of luck that in 2019 I visited the Paris exposition *Le Modèle Noir* and came to terms with the notion that the Black model in Parisian art had been a troublesome theme. Yes, Black models had been present in the history of art, but unidentified, in a certain sense unrecognized, and certainly unknown. Through repeated perusal of the accompanying program catalogue (Musée d'Orsay 2019), I began to comprehend better this problem of invisibility in art history. Or at least, I appreciated its complexity more and grasped that the notion of invisibility may be seen from different angles.

Also in 2019, I had the experience of touring a restored plantation house in the Caribbean and came across the small, recessed room at the back of a regular bedroom. I was told that those rooms were often used to hide away psychiatric patients whom families wished to keep hidden from visitors. Then, later that year, I visited Paris's Sainte-Anne Psychiatric Hospital and learned about the collection of art in the hospital's files. Sainte-Anne was working to make their collection and their artist-patients more visible too. In *Le Modèle Noir*, while maintaining a focus on the profession of Black modeling in Parisian art, emphasis was also placed on the relative absence of Black figures in 19th-century French art. In addition, commentators noted that it was difficult to precisely ascertain the history and sociology of Blacks in Parisian culture. Indeed, the value and meaning of Blackness in French culture at the beginning of the 20th century became intriguingly opaque.

The lack of clarity was even more evident in the years after World War II when exiled American Black individuals in Paris seemed to be accepted more readily than African Black people and individuals from the Maghreb. France's history as a European imperialist power and participant in enslavement was full of contradictions. Nevertheless, I am left with the feeling that although Black models in French art became progressively more visible, I would not assert that Black persons as a general matter have acquired sufficient voice and influence in France and the United States for us to conclude that the problem of visibility has been solved.

On both sides of the Atlantic in the 1930s and 1940s, there was a troubling sort of invisibility of Black people. That is why Suzanne and Aimé Césaire, like others, both raised their voices within the negritude movement in 1930s Paris. Still, looking at Suzanne Césaire's life story, particularly after she returned to Martinique, it is hard to conclude that she was successful in claiming voice. New York's Harlem Renaissance also flowered in the 1920s and 1930s, as writers, painters, sculptors, and photographers found visibility.

The Spanish psychiatrist Francesc Tosquelles was also concerned, around World War II, about the invisibility of psychiatric patients, hidden behind hospital walls that kept them away from the nearby community. Tosquelles started a movement that urged a change from considering psychiatric patients as anonymous beings to viewing them as visible persons with status and dignity. This transformation required patients to contribute in some fashion both to the asylum and to the surrounding community. It was a way of gaining status, purpose, and eventual influence. It involved manifesting oneself, witnessing to having been present at some community happening or other. Artists, when so disposed, can competently make sure that a model, Black or not, is present in a particular landscape. When that happens, the acknowledged appearance becomes a form of testimonial presence. This role was played to the hilt by photographers during the Harlem Renaissance (The Studio Museum in Harlem; Miers 1987).

Over the years, my reflections about invisibility have brought me to recognize how the mechanism of invisibility-rendering may be used within work settings and different landscapes. I suspect that this familiarity with the invisibility phenomenon was aided by the publication of Ralph Ellison's *Invisible Man* (Ellison 1952). In my early clinical experience, I heard clinicians' complaints of being rendered invisible within the group. Some members of a clinical team complained of not being seen and respected by the supervisor, who during extended time periods resorted to rendering a team member invisible within the group. The process involved avoiding use of that person's name, rarely looking in her direction, and minimizing opportunities for her to speak. Those were simple ways of making the person unknown to the group and uncertain of her own identity and value. An obviously different set of interactions could readily have converted that individual from uncertain, hesitant membership into vibrant participation and valued attachment to colleagues. Visibility by itself may not always be sufficient to provoke satisfaction, at least not for extended periods of time. Certainly, in the case of superior athletes, a good relationship with the audience is necessary to help sustain the superathletes' views of themselves as valuable commodities and special entertainment artists. Even a minor injury can provoke thoughts of unworthiness.

Our flamenco artist in this chapter continued pursuing what he called "the art of being," making himself visible through his artistic performances and developing an identity. One may hypothesize that in his efforts to establish himself as an accomplished musician, he was also engaged in constructing a settled inner core of confidence. In other words, thinking about this brilliant musician made me realize that within any geographic space is the passive operation of individuals being rendered invisible by others. Simultaneously, however, some individuals take a back seat and withdraw from the act of rendering themselves visible.

That was not the situation of the flamenco guitarist. After making the move from his home country to overseas, he wished to introduce his genre of music to citizens in this new country. (Here, for simplicity's sake, I put aside the separate notion of involuntary exile, which has its own major complexities.) The task of introducing flamenco music to foreign audiences was enlarged by the need to set up a new home, build a family, and handle all the intricacies of acculturating to a new land. In trying to follow what he meant by pursuing the art of being, I recognized his wish to explain to his audiences why his music was so fundamentally important in the broad scheme of his life course. He would do so by explaining his music's long developmental history and its connections to other cultures and other musical traditions. I tried to put myself in his place when he was playing his guitar. His performance was so earnest, intense, and thoroughly rehearsed that the beauty of each note and the exquisite nature of the performance worked its own magic to force the audience to acknowledge his art. He was a class act. There was no question about that.

Having explored the mechanism of visibility as a means of attaining identity and freedom, in both a personal and an artistic sense, I turn now to reflecting on the notion of self-exile. I also anticipate readers' questions about voluntary or self-imposed exile. Josenhans (2017) explored the connections between forced exile and art in an edited collection of essays. Forced displacement has powerful examples in the movement of Jewish artists from Nazi Germany to safety elsewhere. That form of massive, mandated upheaval is not my focus here.

William Gardner Smith (1963/2021) saw the forms of voluntary exile mentioned here as a form of geographic displacement, political activism, and quest for freedom—as in the movement of Black migrants from the South to the North of the United States and in the displacement of Black American artists from the United States to France in the 1940s and 1950s. The Windrush movement of Caribbean people from the West Indies to Britain in the 1950s is another example. These movements had as objectives, besides obvious economic interests, the building of identity, the acquisition of self-respect, and the enjoyment of a sense of emancipation.

Hilton Als (1998) described James Baldwin's taking leave of the United States in 1948, partly to escape the disenfranchisement of his early life in the United States and to fulfill his promised identity as a literary artist. It was a move that Richard Wright, Sidney Bechet, Josephine Baker, and many others had also made. Als reported that Baldwin was just beginning to taste some recognition as a writer when he made his move to Paris. He also pointed out that Baldwin, in eventually gaining success, would still have to settle scores with his unknown biological father, his adoptive father, and his paternal artistic supporter in Richard Wright. In other words, there is more involved in making a geographic move than simply executing the act of changing one's residence. The process of acculturating to the new place is a major task, as is also the act of setting up a new home. Seeking freedom is no simplistic task.

Over the last decade or so, the political implications of migrating to Europe have been captured in many a debate. Some politicians have tried to quantify the degree of change an immigrant must make on arriving in the host country. Mandatory changes might include the type of clothes worn by the children to school, or by the adult women, and enforced religious practices or ways of raising children. Discussions of these ideas raise questions about which aspects of migration are voluntary or involuntary and which dimensions of acculturation might be expected to evoke protest or resistance from the immigrant families. This conversation has taken place in countries where the central problem has been the division within the country of whether to pursue a genuinely multicultural society or a more nationalistic unicultural orientation. In the latter context, mandates related to dress, education, language, and religion seem to be more commonly encountered.

Two columns in this chapter, one focused on the solitude of an artist and the other concerning a potter, contemplate a unique approach to the artist's search for freedom. The first story describes a pianist who developed a successful career as a musician and had a penchant for privacy and a sense of independence about how to execute his art. From early, he enjoyed personal isolation, eventually even from his audiences, family, and close friends, while maintaining an interest in how he executed his art and defined his distinctive aesthetic. As presented in the play about his life, it seemed to me that his conceptualization of freedom was attuned mostly to his professional and personal life. He wished to function in a bubble that he defined and controlled. He seemed to have little interest in a community construct of freedom.

In the case of the potter, he was pleased with the palpable peacefulness of his work, but in our discussions made clear that in his art he was not connected to any social movement. He represented himself and saw freedom as embodied in the execution of his sculptures. He did not want his art to convey any special message from him, one that was distinguishable from the process of his artistic creativity. It is striking how different these two artists were from the members of the Harlem Renaissance. As I discussed in the column "Talkin' 'Bout Harlem" earlier in this chapter, the Black artists of that period saw their artistic work as interrogating commentaries on sexuality, homophobia, racism, colorism, and cultural solidarity. Similarly, in the column "Yonder on the Other Side," the theme of the play was related to the problem of European colonization and freedom in the context of the relationship between Algeria and France.

The column concerning the manifestation of ancestral dignity and the other one dealing with Suzanne Césaire and Caribbean identity have some intriguing commonalities. The former, rooted in Barbados, emerged from that small Anglophone island-nation's efforts to manage its emergence from colonization by Great Britain and the decision to become a new republic. Facing independence, the island's citizens settled on the construction of Freedom Park and Builders of Barbados Wall. The intent was to memorialize the contributions Barbadians made to the survival of the island's dignity throughout time. Artists transformed the park and wall into a unique area representing a collective public monument to ancestral dignity. The column I wrote about Suzanne Césaire's search for a Martiniquan identity documented her interest in a similar national scheme for her island. She articulated her ideas of native independence well before the end of World War II, grounding it in the Caribbean, and explicitly on the backs of generations of women in whom she had faith. She was seeking self-acknowledgment, but for everyone on the island.

It is curious that I started my journey in Barbados contemplating life as defined by an Anglophone imperialism. Then, after taking different roads, I returned to the Caribbean reflecting on what a feminist philosopher suggested about the task of seeking freedom, independence of spirit, and an identity both personal and harnessed to professional formation. I have come to accept that who I am cannot be linked uniquely to other people's ideas of me. Their formulation of my worth and value and their attribution of dignity to me as a person cannot unilaterally define me. I must emerge from my own struggles to work things out, to define who and what can be trusted.

As I pointed out in the column on Suzanne Césaire, she did not accept others' vision of Martinique as a bucolic land waiting to provide pleasure submissively to others. She wanted to achieve confidence in herself and her ancestors. That did not mean she wished to deny what France and Africa could teach her about the complexity of life. In fact, she acknowledged that she would learn things from many of the countries proximate to Martinique, including the United States. However, she did not wish to bind herself slavishly to imitating others. Martinique had its own history, traditions, and pride. With the requisite self-confidence, she could build on what she learned from her own past and from others and produce a future full of hope and dignity.

## Questions to Ponder

1. Whether to render a patient's psychiatric disability visible is a knotty problem. Is it the patient's choice, or should the health system take a firm position on this?
2. What is your view of using violence to protest discrimination?
3. Should governments allow the use of public spaces for protest art by its citizens?
4. Should we support artists whose only intent is to stay within the boundaries of aesthetics?
5. Do you have any idea of the criteria needed to define Black art of the Harlem Renaissance? Can a White artist authentically represent that art?

## References

Als H: The enemy within: the making and unmaking of James Baldwin. New Yorker, February 16, 1998

Bernal MC: A voice for surrealism: Suzanne Césaire and the Tropiques group. Int J Surrealism 1(1):40–57, 2023

Chambers V, May-Curry M: The dinner party that started the Harlem Renaissance. New York Times, March 21, 2024

Cotter H: The Met aims to get Harlem right, the second time around. New York Times, February 19, 2024

Ellison R: Invisible Man. New York, Random House, 1952

Hannaham J: A Black writer found tolerance in France, and a different racism. New York Times, July 19, 2021

Josenhans FV (ed): Artists in Exile: Expressions of Loss and Hope. New Haven, CT, Yale University Art Gallery, 2017

McKay C: Home to Harlem. New York, Harper & Brothers, 1928

Meier A: Harlem is now truly on the Met's mind. Art Newspaper, February 20, 2024

Miers C (ed): Harlem Renaissance: Art of Black America. Studio Museum in Harlem. New York, Harry N. Abrams Publishers, 1987

Musée d'Orsay: Le Modèle Noir De Géricault À Matisse. Paris, Musée d'Orsay/Flammarion, 2019

Rabbitt K: The geography of identity in Suzanne Césaire's "Le grand camouflage." Res Afr Lit 39(3):121–131, 2008

Saïd G: Suzanne Césaire, la poésie en partage. Diacritik, April 18, 2016

Smith WG: The Stone Face. Chicago, IL, Farrar, Straus, 1963; reprinted New York, New York Review of Books Classics, 2021

# Epilogue

It is finished, the documenting of the tale about my wanderings between 2019 and 2024. It has been a remarkable experience contemplating the many people I have held conversations with, and in the most interesting of places, about the subjects considered by them to be important. I have been able to recount in this text only a fraction of my experiences along the way. Nevertheless, I confirmed several ideas or principles that I developed over time. For example, I realized that the expression noted by some—that life is storied—is real and intriguing. A university reunion I attended only a month ago bore witness to that notion. I simply stood still with some practiced patience while old friends plied me with accounts of the strangest and most intimate of events. In this text, I have made use of narratives about many subjects and in a particularly brief format. I hope you have found it worth your time and effort.

Coming to the end of this experience brings to mind conversations with Dr. Miraj Desai, at the time a young Yale University colleague. We discussed the values of travel in improving scholarship and clinical work. His point was that travel-inspired observation and reflection may well ameliorate clinical insight and therapeutic technique. He told me about the possibility of promoting openness and contemplative awareness in the process of engaging with different cultures and people. Like me, he had experienced growing up in a culture, then confronting the feelings generated by movement into other societies. At the heart of this process has been, at every turn, the effort required to confront difference: to see it, feel it, evaluate it if necessary, and respect the reality that it is not our familiar sameness. Still, it deserves our respect and consideration, with acknowledgment that difference in people, especially, should not reflexively evoke our sense of superiority.

# Index

Page numbers printed in **boldface** type refer to tables or figures.

16th-Century Altarpiece, A, Colmar, France, **123**
1990 Americans With Disabilities Act, 66

Adshead, Gwen, 41–42
Affirmative action, 39–40
*African American Bioethics: Culture, Race, and Identity*, 2
African American studies, 24
Age and politics, 177–179, 181
Algerian War, 194, **195**
  Algerian National Liberation Front, 194, **195**
Altarpiece, 122, **123**, 124
  images of the, 124
American Academy of Psychiatry and the Law, 32
*American Heritage Dictionary*, 163
American Medical Association, 3
American Psychiatric Association (APA), 2, 5, 74
  Annual Meeting in 2019, 2–3
  Black members of, 5
*Analytical Concordance to the Bible*, 166
Anglican Church, 21, 37, 57, 98, **131**
Archiving, 165–169, 182
Art brut, 84
*Artists in Exile: Expressions of Loss and Hope*, 105
*At War With the Obvious: Disruptive Thinking in Psychoanalysis*, 81

*Ballad of Suzanne Césaire, The*, 207, 209
Barbadian Moravian church, 134
Barbadian music, 99, 124, 146
  pan music, 126
  steel pan concerts, 100
  steel pan movement, 124, 126
  Tamboo-Bamboo musical groups, 124

Barbadian outfits, 98
Basilica Sant'Andrea (Basilica of St. Andrew), 139, **140**
Béguerie-De Paepe, Pantxika, 122
"Being and Blackness," 4
*Belonging, Therapeutic Landscapes, and Networks*, xxxii
*Beyond a Boundary*, 160–161, 182
Bioethics, 3
Biomedical psychiatry, xxviii
*Black Is the Color of My Voice*, 191
Black Power moment, 37
Black Psychiatrists of America, 42
Blacks, 2–5, 142–150
  in Barbados, 21–22
  Blackness, 4
  discrimination against, 2
  law enforcement by police on, 12
  mental health of, 3
  models in French art, 210
  patients' rights and privileges, 3
  rights and privileges, 5
Black solidarity, 4
*Blueprint: The Evolutionary Origins of a Good Society*, 3
Bohemia Reformation, 134
*Book of Jesse, The*, 135
Brooks, Peter, 40
*Brothers Karamazov, The*, 82
Bubonic plague, 107
Burke, Vanley, 49, 58

Caribbean, 21
  celebration of native heroes, 35
  colonialism in, 21
  cuisine, 22
  home-space, 22
  immigrants in New York City, 24

Caste, 130
  and othering, 130
  othering by United States and Russia, 130
*Caste: The Origins of Our Discontents*, 8, 27, 130
Césaire, Suzanne, 207–210, 214–215
Champs Élysées, xxxiii, 112
Chauvin, Derek, 10, 13, 55
  Chauvin verdict, 14, 27
  police brutality, 27
Cherry blossom tree music festival, 109, **111**
Chéry, Jacques Richard, 77, **78**
Christakis, Nicholas, 3
  social suite concept, 4
Clinical observations, 21–27, 53–60, 87–93, 114–119, 145–150, 180–182, 210–215
Colonial oppression, 60
  in Algeria, xxx
  European and American, 25
A Common Ritual at Weddings in Morocco, **54**
Community mental health center (CMHC) movement, 89
Compassion, 32, 56, 117
  defined, 32
Contagion, 100–101, 109
  literature of, 116
  prevention of, 117
*Contemporary Psychoanalysis*, 6
Coronavirus disease 2019 (COVID-19), 6, 68, 101, 108, 115, 127
  belief in God, 116
  Capuchin monks, 102, 115
  concerns of vulnerability, 105
  feelings of believers, 102
  as fracture in human connections, 117
  home as space during, 103
  isolation and abandonment, 117–118
  psychological distance, 106
  reaction to suffering, 102
  resurrection and renewal, 118
  stories of epidemics, 100
Culture-bound gatherings, 79
  end-of-year rituals, 91
  end-of-year season, 80
Curiosity about the other, 12, 16–17
Czech Republic, 134

Davidson, Larry, 88–90
Death and religion, 114–115, 118
*Diacritik*, 207
Dignity, 33, 51, 53, 55, 58, 70, 77, 142
  attributed, 33, 53
  case of George Floyd, 55
  defined, 53
  immigration problem, 142
  intrinsic, 33, 53, 56
  loss of identity or status, 59
  memorializing of, 57
  in physical looks and clothing, 146
  in public monuments, 201–202
    Builders of Barbados Wall, **204**
    Clement Payne Statue, **203**
  racialized discrimination, 59
Dignity and identity, 34, 161
Disabilities, 64, 91
  deaf militancy, 65
  deafness, 64–65, 87
  isolation, 64
Disciplinary power, 9
Discrimination, xxxii, xxxiii
  race-based, 4
Displacement and mobility, 23
Diversity, 2, 16, 26
  12 principles of, 16
  biopower, 26
  competency and literacy, 16
Dubois, Anne Marie, 187

Empathy, 32, 56
  defined, 32
Ethiopian classical music, 51–52
Ethiopian Orthodox Church, 52
Ethnocultural consciousness, xxix
An Exemplar of *Stolpersteine* in Berlin, **8**

Fanon, Frantz, 85
*Fire Next Time, The*, 10
Flamenco dance, **191**, 191–192, 212
Floyd, George, 10, 14–15, 55
Forensic psychiatry, 32
  pursuit of objectivity and truth, 32
Forgiveness, 80–82, 91
Foucault, Michel, 9
Francesc (François) Tosquelles: Avant-Garde Psychiatry and the Birth of Art Brut, 83
Freedom, 17–19
*Free World: Art and Thought in the Cold War, The*, 18

*Index*

*Freud et la Femme de Chambre* (*Freud and the Housekeeper*), 175–177
Freud, Sigmund, 175–177, 181
   on God's existence, 176

Gatherin', 98, 100, 119
Geller, Jeffrey, 5
Geographic/pyschological distance, 118
Geography and health, 154
George Floyd Justice in Policing Act (HR 7120), 15
*Glenn: Birth of a Prodigy* (*Glenn: Naissance d'un Prodige*), 196–197
Gould, Glenn, 196–197
Grantham, Ronald, 198
   life and art of, 198–199, **200**
Guédiguian, Robert, 159
Gutenberg Bible, 163

Haas, Magali, 122
Hagenauer, Nikolaus, 122
Harlem Renaissance, 205–206, 211
*Harlem Renaissance: Art of Black America*, 205–206
Hart, Anton, 16–17
*Harvard Gazette, The*, 14
Haydn, Franz Joseph, 80
Hickling, Frederick, 7, 19, 38
   European-American psychosis, 7
Hiroshima bombings, 127
Hogan, Eileen, 154
   public parks, 155
Holy Eucharist, xxxiii
Home-space(s), 154, 160, 180–181
*Home to Harlem*, 206
*House by the Sea, The*, 159–160, 181
Human flourishing, 3
Hunt-Ehrlich, Madeleine, 207–208

Identity, 37
Idowu, Joel Akande, 45–46, **47**, 48
*I'm Your Father, Boy*, xxxiii
Indignity, 53, 60
Inequality, 12
*Invisible Man*, 211
Isenheim Altarpiece, 122, **123**, 148
*Isenheim Altarpiece, The*, 122
Italian Renaissance music, 163, **164**, 165

James, Cyril Lionel Robert, 161, 183

Kafka, Franz, 135, 138
Kathleen, Young, 6
King, Martin Luther, 18, 25
   equality and freedom, 19
"Knee on the Other's Neck, The," xxxii, 10–15
Koz, Gabriel, **73**, 74–75

Lincoln Hospital in New York City, 72, 74–75, 89
Loss and hope, 103, 105

Malcolm X, 25
Marin, Claire, 117–119
Martinez, Daniel, 191, 193
Mbappé, Kylian, 189
Menand, Louis, 18
Mental health, 40
Mental illness, 66
*Metamorphosis, The*, 135
Metropolitan Museum of Art, 142, 144, 204
   *Harlem on My Mind*, 205
   *Harlem Renaissance and Transatlantic Modernism*, 204
Moore, Dougles, 80
Moss, Donald, 81–82
*Mother and Daughter*, 207
Musée d'Art et d'Histoire de l'Hôpital Sainte-Anne (MAHHSA), 69, 187, **188**
   La Maison-Hôpital, 70
   A l'Intérieur de l'Intime, 70
   as place of healthful restoration, 71
   Rêve d'Habitation, 71
   Vers La Demeure, 70

National Association for the Advancement of Colored People, 206
*Native Son*, 24
Nelson, Vice Adm. Lord Horatio, 34–35
New Negro movement, 205
New Testament, 108
   Matthew, 108, 133
*New Yorker, The*, 18
*New York Times, The*, 14, 17
Nithart, Mathis Gothart, 122
Norko, Michael, 39
Nostalgia, 118
Notre Dame Cathedral, 101, **102**

Old Testament, 107
    Leviticus, 107
"On Caste and Suffering," xxxii, 8–10
Open Door Christian Church, 102
*Organization and Delivery of Mental Health Services in the Ghetto: The Lincoln Hospital Experience, The*, 75

Pasteur Institute in Saigon, 107, 112
Patient advocacy, xxviii
Pellegrino, Edmund, 2–3
*People's History of Psychoanalysis, A*, 45
Personal restorative power, 100
Philharmonic Society of St. Petersburg, 129, **130**
Photography and memory, 172–174
Piazza Erbe, 138–139, **139**
Pierce, Chester, 3
Place and health, 154–155, 181
    Danielle-Mitterrand garden, 155, **156**
    healing environment, 154
    mental illnesses and home communities, 154
    public gardens, 156–158
Plague of leprosy, 107
Political activism, 14
Political independence, 37, 57
Pragmatic nationalism, 4
"Principles of Teaching Issues of Diversity in a Psychoanalytic Context," 16
*Prodigal, The*, 35
*Psychiatric News* (American Psychiatric Association), xxvii, xxxv
Psychiatric rehabilitation, 67, 70, 76, 92
    rehabilitation, 69
*Psychiatric Services*, 75
Psychosocial experience(s), xxvii
Public Monument on the Seine River, Paris, France, **195**

Quai Branly Jacques Chirac Museum, 193

*Race and Excellence*, 104
Racism, xxxii
    anti-Black violence, 14
    race and caste, 25
    racial hatred, 6–7
    racialized thinking and discourse, 26
    racial self-hatred, 7
"Raconte-moi ta vieillesse," 177
Recovery, 66, 88, 90
Recreating home, 190–192
Religion, 127
    acceptance of the, 144
    and activities in secular spheres, 145
    churchgoing in Barbados, 145
    and colonial oppression, 144
    personal suffering, 133
    sacred spaces, 145–146, 148–149
    service to others, 128
Rock Hall Monument of Freedom, The, **20**
Rowling, J. K., 186
Royal Processional Route, 132
Russian church music, 129–130, 148

Sainte-Anne Psychiatric Hospital in Paris, 68, 186–187, 210
Salovey, Peter, 13
Sculpture of Franz Kafka's Head by David Černý, **136–137**
Secondary decolonization, 37–38
Slave Code of 1661, 57
Smith, Quentin Ted, 42, **43**, 45
Smith, William Gardner, 194, 212
Smyth, Fiona, 180
Social justice, 2
Solidarity, 115
St. Anthony, 122–123
    image in the altarpiece, 122
St. Anthony's Fire, 122
Statue of William Lanson by Dana King, **36**
Steel Pan Concert at St. James Parish Church, **125**
St. John's Scottish Episcopal Church, 126–127
*Stone Face, The*, 193
Stress, 189–190
    commitment, 190
    sports performance, 189–190
St. Sebastian, 123
"Surviving Hating and Being Hated: Some Personal Thoughts About Racism From a Psychoanalytic Perspective," 6

# Index

Task Force to Address Structural Racism Throughout Psychiatry, 5
*Testimony*, xxxv
Tosquelles, Francesc, 83–85, 89
Trump, Donald, xxviii

Venice International Film Festival, 74th, 159
Vietnam War, 114
Virgin Mary, 123
Visibility, 186–187
"Visibility in a Psychiatric Hospital's Museum," 68
Vltava River, 134
Vocation, 39–40

Wagner, Richard, 79
Walcott, Derek, 105
War and misery, 111–113
*Webster's Universal Dictionary*, 166

*We Who Are Dark: The Philosophical Foundations of Black Solidarity*, 4
"When Diversity Is Not Enough," 2–3, 26
White, Kathleen, 7
White privilege, 7
White superiority, 38
White supremacy, 35
Whitney Plantation of Louisiana, The, **13**
Wilkerson, Isabel, 9
  caste, 9, 24
  medical caste system, 9–10
Williams, Francis, 49
Williams, Granville, 143, 148
Workspace(s), 180, 182

Yale Beinecke Rare Book and Manuscript Library, 163, **164**, 182
*Ye Shall Dream*, xxxiv, 142
Yifrashewa, Girma, 51–52

9798894551401